Applied Radiological Anatomy

This helpful revision aid will be of great practical benefit to all trainees in radiology, including those studying the new modular curriculum for Fellowship of the Royal College of Radiologists Part 2A examination. The carefully structured questions and answers enable the trainees to undertake a systematic assessment of their knowledge, as well as highlighting areas where additional revision is required. This publication has been designed to complement its highly illustrated companion volume *Applied Radiological Anatomy* (by Butler, Mitchell & Ellis), which itself serves as a comprehensive overview of anatomy as illustrated by the full range of modern radiological procedures. Both books can be used independently of one another; however, it is anticipated that the trainee will gain maximum benefit from using the two books together. Although allied closely to the curriculum for the new radiology exam, the choice of questions will be relevant and useful for radiology trainees world-wide.

Arockia Doss is Specialist Registrar in the Department of Radiology of the Royal Hallamshire Hospital at the Sheffield Teaching Hospitals NHS Trust, UK

Matthew J. Bull is Consultant Radiologist and Program Director of the North Trent Radiology Training Scheme of the Sheffield Teaching Hospitals NHS Trust at the Northern General Hospital in Sheffield, UK

Alan Sprigg is Consultant Radiologist in X-ray and Imaging at the Sheffield Children's Hospital at the Sheffield Teaching Hospitals NHS Trust, UK

Paul D. Griffiths is Professor of Radiology in the Section of Academic Radiology of the Department of Radiology at the Royal Hallamshire Hospital at the Sheffield Teaching Hospitals NHS Trust, UK

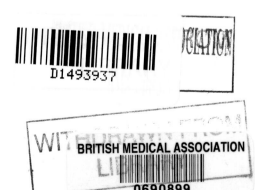

MCQ Companion to

Applied Radiological Anatomy

Arockia Doss, Matthew J. Bull
Alan Sprigg and Paul D. Griffiths

Sheffield Teaching Hospitals NHS Trust, UK

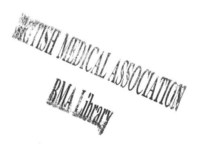

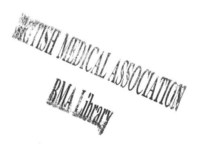

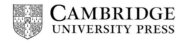
CAMBRIDGE
UNIVERSITY PRESS

PUBLISHED BY THE PRESS SYNDICATE OF THE UNIVERSITY OF CAMBRIDGE
The Pitt Building, Trumpington Street, Cambridge, United Kingdom

CAMBRIDGE UNIVERSITY PRESS
The Edinburgh Building, Cambridge CB2 2RU, UK
40 West 20th Street, New York, NY 10011–4211, USA
477 Williamstown Road, Port Melbourne, VIC 3207, Australia
Ruiz de Alarcón 13, 28014 Madrid, Spain
Dock House, The Waterfront, Cape Town 8001, South Africa

http://www.cambridge.org

First published 2003

Printed in the United Kingdom at the University Press, Cambridge

Typeface Utopia 9.5/13 pt   *System* QuarkXPress™   [SE]

A catalogue record for this book is available from the British Library

Library of Congress Cataloguing in Publication data

MCQ companion to Applied radiological anatomy: preparation for the modules of FRCR 2A /
Arockia Doss . . . [et al.].
    p. ; cm.
Includes bibliographical references and index.
ISBN 0 521 52153 X (pb.)
1. Radiography, Medical – Examinations, questions, etc.   2. Human anatomy –
Examinations, questions, etc.   I. Doss, Arockia, 1970–
II. Applied radiological anatomy.
[DNLM: 1. Anatomy – Examination Questions.   2. Radiology – Examination Questions.
QS 18.2 M478 2003]
RC78 .A675 1999 Suppl.
616.07′572′076 – dc21   2002025688

ISBN 0 521 52153 X paperback

To my Dad and wife Josephin
who always gave me the best   AD

To Amanda, Charlotte, Emily and Lydia

MJB

Contents

Foreword

It is a pleasure to write a Foreword to this book of MCQs. Sometimes an 'accompanying volume' is a poor relation of the original; not this one – it made me thirst to go to the excellent original to check and recheck my (rusty) facts!

It is also pleasing to see an MCQ book entirely devoted to radiological anatomy. Many medical schools are currently reducing the content of their anatomy (morphology, architecture, etc.) courses, given perceived overloading of the curriculum. Thus future radiological trainees may have less background anatomical knowledge than their predecessors. Radiology depends entirely on being able to recognise normal anatomy, anatomical variants thereof and abnormal structures. Indeed, detailed knowledge of anatomy and applied techniques is usually the deciding characteristic among radiologists and clinicians with an interest in imaging. It behoves all radiologists to learn anatomy in depth and to maintain and develop that knowledge throughout their professional career.

This book also serves as a reminder to examination candidates (and examiners) that anatomical questions are still very much in vogue within the new Royal College of Radiologists' examination scheme. This book jumps ahead so that the questions are grouped together in system-based modules: a forerunner of things to come.

Setting MCQs is no easy task. The authors have done a good job to make them relevant and realistic for examination purposes. Of course, there will be one or two minor quibbles when the book is reviewed and most statements including 'may' are true! However, this is not the point. This is a revision (or in some cases a vision) for those working to attain a certain standard of radiological anatomical knowledge. To this end, this slim volume will be an enormous help and even makes for an amusing brain exercise for more senior citizens. I congratulate the authors and hope that the book gains the success it deserves.

Adrian K. Dixon
July 2002

Preface

One of the best ways to prepare well for an MCQ exam is to make up MCQs whilst reading a text. This book is the result of such an effort for the Fellowship of the Royal College of Radiologists (FRCR) 1 exam with the textbook *Applied Radiological Anatomy*.

The Royal College of Radiologists recently introduced the modular exam for the FRCR 2A. The radiological anatomy, techniques and physics will contribute about 15–20% of all the MCQs. The purpose of this work is to present questions on radiological anatomy for the six modules of the FRCR 2A. Therefore, the book is presented as six modules, each representing a module for the FRCR 2A. The modules should be read in conjunction with chapters in the textbook *Applied Radiological Anatomy*. The questions with the relevant answers are on opposite pages which makes easy reading. Some questions are based on pathology and some are related to general radiological technique from day-to-day practice. It is hoped that this will be stimulating to the trainee and help with better understanding in acquiring the general skills of performing and reporting radiological examinations.

We have not included a separate module on surface anatomy. However, questions on relevant surface anatomy are included in the various modules. Some of the chapters from *Applied Radiological Anatomy* have been included in a related module. For example, the chapter on renal tract and retroperitoneum and pelvis has been included in Module 4.

It is hoped that this book will provide radiology trainees with a focused approach to learning MCQs from different anatomical locations and prepare them well for the modules of the FRCR 2A.

AD, MJB, AS, PDG
Sheffield, UK
January 2002

Acknowledgements

AD is indebted to Drs M. J. Bull, A. Sprigg and Professor P. D. Griffiths, as this book would not have been possible without them. AD is also grateful to Drs Michael C. Collins, Robert J. Peck, Richard Nakielny, Christine Davies, Tony Blakeborough, and all Consultant Radiologists of the Sheffield Teaching Hospitals NHS Trust, Sheffield, UK, whose teachings have been included in the text. AD would also like to thank Peter Silver in the publications department for his support and enthusiasm. We thank all our families for their patience during the preparation of this book. We also thank Liz and Jane at the Northern General Hospital, Sheffield, for the preparation of the manuscript.

Module 1

Chest and cardiovascular

A. Doss and M. J. Bull

1. Regarding the imaging modalities of the chest:

(a) High resolution computed tomography (HRCT) uses a slice thickness of 4–6 mm to identify mass lesions in the lung.
(b) Spiral CT ensures that no portion of the chest is missed due to variable inspiratory effort.
(c) MRI shows excellent detail of the lung anatomy.
(d) Bronchography is the technique of choice to visualize the bronchial tree
(e) CT pulmonary angiography (CTPA) is performed using catheters placed in a femoral vein.

2. Regarding the development of the lung:

(a) The tracheobronchial groove appears on the ventral aspect of the caudal end of the pharynx.
(b) The primary bronchial buds develop from the tracheobronchial diverticulum.
(c) The epithelium lining the alveoli is the same before and after birth.
(d) A persistent tracheo-oesophageal fistula (TOF) is commonly associated with an atresia of the duodenum.
(e) Uni-lateral pulmonary hypoplasia is usually due to a congenital diaphragmatic hernia.

3. Regarding the blood supply to the chest wall:

(a) The posterior intercostal arteries supply the 11 intercostal spaces.
(b) The internal thoracic artery arises from the subclavian artery and supplies the upper six intercostal spaces.
(c) The neurovascular bundle passes around the chest wall in the subcostal groove deep to the internal intercostal muscle.

Chest and cardiovascular

ANSWERS

1.

(a) False – HRCT uses 1–2 mm slice thickness and a high resolution computer algorithm to show fine detail of the lung parenchyma, pleura and tracheobronchial tree. It is not used to delineate masses in the lung.

(b) True

(c) False – currently MRI is a poor technique for showing lung detail. It allows visualisation of the chest wall, heart, mediastinal and hilar structures.

(d) False – this invasive technique has largely been superseded by HRCT.

(e) False – CTPA is performed to diagnose major pulmonary emboli using a cannula placed in any peripheral vein and is relatively non-invasive compared to conventional pulmonary angiography.

2.

(a) True

(b) True – the bronchial buds differentiate into bronchi in each lung.

(c) False – during embryonic life the alveoli is lined by cuboidal epithelium that lines the rest of the respiratory tract. When respiration commences at birth the transfer to the flattened pavement epithelium of the alveoli is accomplished.

(d) False – TOF indicates the close developmental relationship between the foregut and the respiratory passages. It is usually associated with an atresia of the oesophagus and the fistula is situated below the atretic segment.

(e) True

3.

(a) False – there are usually nine pairs of posterior arteries from the postero-lateral margin of the thoracic aorta, distributed to the lower nine intercostal spaces. The first and second spaces are supplied by the superior intercostal artery, branches of the costocervical trunk from the subclavian artery.

(b) True

(c) True

(d) The intercostal spaces are drained by two anterior veins and a single posterior intercostal vein.
(e) The posterior intercostal vein drains into the internal thoracic vein.

4. Regarding the azygos venous system:

(a) The azygos vein at the level of the fourth thoracic vertebra arches over the root of the right lung to end in the superior vena cava (SVC).
(b) About 10% of the population have an azygos lobe.
(c) The thoracic duct and aorta are to the right of the azygos vein.
(d) The second, third and fourth intercostal spaces on the right, drain via the right superior intercostal vein into the azygos vein.
(e) In congenital absence of IVC the azygos vein enlarges.

5. Regarding the hemiazygos and accessory hemiazygos venous systems:

(a) The hemiazygos vein at the level of the fourth thoracic vertebra crosses the vertebral column behind the aorta, oesophagus and thoracic duct.
(b) The ascending lumbar veins and the lower three posterior intercostal veins are the tributaries of the hemiazygos vein.
(c) The accessory hemiazygos vein receives the fourth to the eighth intercostal veins on the left.
(d) The accessory hemiazygos vein may drain into the left brachiocephalic vein.
(e) The first posterior intercostal vein may drain into the corresponding vertebral vein.

6. Regarding the airways:

(a) In adults the right main-stem bronchus is steeper than the left.
(b) The left main bronchus is about twice as long as the right.
(c) The bronchioles contain cartilage.
(d) Gas exchange takes place in the terminal bronchioles and acini.
(e) The bronchopulmonary segments are based on the pulmonary arterial system.

(d) True
(e) False – posterior intercostal veins drain into the brachiocephalic vein and azygos system. The anterior veins drain into the musculo-phrenic and internal thoracic veins.

4.

(a) True
(b) False – in 1% of the population, the azygos vein traverses the lung before entering the SVC resulting in the azygos fissure. The azygos ' lobe' is not a true segment.
(c) False – they are to its left.
(d) True – hemiazygos, accessory hemiazygos, oesophageal, mediastinal, pericardial and right bronchial veins drain into the azygos system.
(e) True – in the azygous continuation of the IVC, the azygos is a large structure, but otherwise the anatomy is unaltered. This may be confused with a mediastinal mass.

5.

(a) False – at the level of T8.
(b) True – and subcostal veins of the left side, some mediastinal and oesophageal veins.
(c) True – sometimes the bronchial veins.
(d) True – through the left superior intercostal vein. It may join the hemiazygos and/or drain into the azygos vein at the level of T7.
(e) True – or the corresponding brachiocephalic vein.

6.

(a) True
(b) True
(c) False – after 6 to 20 divisions the segmental bronchi no longer contain cartilage in their walls and become bronchioles.
(d) False – the terminal bronchiole is the last of the purely conducting airways, beyond which are the gas-exchange units of the lung – the acini.
(e) False – based on the divisions of the bronchi.

7. Regarding the secondary pulmonary lobule:

(a) It consists of approximately ten acini.
(b) The lobular vein follows the branches of the bronchioles.
(c) Lymph drainage is both interlobular and central along the arteries.
(d) Lobules are best demonstrated nearer to the hilum of the lung on CT.
(e) The interlobular septa are seen usually on conventional CT.

8. Regarding the pulmonary blood vessels:

(a) The bronchovascular bundle of the secondary pulmonary lobule is demonstrated as a rounded density about 1 cm away from the pleural border on axial CT.
(b) The inferior pulmonary veins draining the lower lobes are more vertical than the lower lobe arteries.
(c) The upper lobe veins lie lateral to the arteries.
(d) In a frontal chest radiograph the artery and bronchus of the anterior segment of the upper lobes are frequently seen end-on.
(e) The left pulmonary artery passes anterior to the left main bronchus.

9. Regarding the pleura:

(a) The parietal pleura is continuous with the visceral pleura at the hilum.
(b) On a PA radiograph the pleura is seen in the costophrenic sulcus.
(c) The parietal pleura is supplied by the pulmonary circulation.
(d) The fissures usually contain a layer of parietal and visceral pleura.
(e) The intercostal stripe is seen on axial CT as a linear opacity of soft tissue density at the intercostal space.

10. Regarding the fissures of the lung:

(a) Complete fissures may be crossed by small bronchovascular structures seen on HRCT.
(b) The oblique fissure separates the upper and lower lobes from the middle lobe on the right.

7.

(a) True – acini are 8–20 mm in diameter and consists of respiratory bronchioles, alveolar ducts and alveoli.
(b) False – the lobular artery follows the branches of the bronchioles. Peripheral veins drain the lobule and run along the interlobular septum.
(c) True
(d) False – lobules are surrounded by connective tissue septa which contain veins and lymphatic vessels, in the lung periphery. Therefore they are best demonstrated in the periphery of the lung.
(e) False – they can just be appreciated on HRCT.

8.

(a) True
(b) False – the opposite is true.
(c) True
(d) True
(e) False – it arches over the left main bronchus and left upper lobe bronchus to descend postero-lateral to the left lower lobe bronchus.

9.

(a) True – and in the inferior pulmonary ligament.
(b) False – the visceral pleura can be seen on a plain radiograph only where it invaginates the lung to form fissures and at the junctional lines.
(c) False – the parietal pleura is supplied by the systemic circulation, and the visceral pleura is supplied by the pulmonary and bronchial circulation.
(d) False – only two layers of visceral pleura.
(e) True – two layers of pleura, extrapleural fat, innermost intercostal muscle and endothoracic fascia.

10.

(a) False – incomplete fissures have parenchymal fusion and small bronchovascular structures.
(b) False – the oblique fissure separates the upper and middle lobes from the lower lobe on the right.

(c) The lateral and medial portion of the oblique fissure are equidistant from the anterior chest wall.

(d) The major fissures appear as a soft tissue linear density from the hilum to the chest wall on standard 10 mm thick CT sections.

(e) The minor fissure separates the right middle lobe from the right lower lobe.

11. Regarding the accessory fissures of the lung:

(a) The azygos fissure results from failure of normal migration of the azygos vein from the chest wall through the lung.

(b) The inferior accessory fissure separates the medial basal segment from the rest of the right lower lobe.

(c) The superior accessory fissure lies above the minor fissure.

(d) A left minor fissure is seen in 10% of frontal radiographs.

(e) The inferior pulmonary ligaments are pleural reflections from the pericardium.

12. Regarding blood supply of the lung:

(a) The left bronchial artery arises from the right bronchial artery.

(b) The deep bronchial veins may end in the left atrium.

(c) The right and left pulmonary arteries are at the same height in the chest.

(d) The right upper lobe pulmonary artery is anterior to the right upper lobe bronchus.

(e) The veins of the upper lobe are posterior to the arteries and bronchi.

(c) False – the oblique fissures follow a gently curving plane. The upper portion faces forward and laterally and the lower portion forwards and medially.

(d) False – the most common appearance is a curvilinear avascular band extending from the hilum to the chest wall, reflecting the lack of vessels in the subcortical zone of the lung. On HRCT, the major fissure appears as a line or a band.

(e) False – the minor fissure separates the anterior segment of the right upper lobe from the right middle lobe.

11.

(a) True – almost always on the right, rarely an analogous fissure may be seen on the left with the accessory hemiazygos or left superior intercostal vein.

(b) True – runs upward and medially towards the hilum, from the medial aspect of the diaphragm.

(c) False – superior accessory fissure separates the superior segment of the lower lobe from the basal segments and is inferior to the minor fissure on the frontal radiograph.

(d) False – left minor fissure seen in 10% of individuals is hardly seen on frontal or lateral radiographs. It separates the lingular segments from the rest of the upper lobe.

(e) False – they are pleural reflections that hang down from the hila and from the mediastinal surface of each lower lobe to the mediastinum and to the medial part of the diaphragm.

12.

(a) False – bronchial arteries are variable. Usually the right bronchial artery arises from the third posterior intercostal artery or from the upper left bronchial artery. The left bronchial arteries are two in number and arise from the thoracic aorta.

(b) True – the deep bronchial veins communicate freely with the pulmonary veins, end in a pulmonary vein or left atrium. The superficial bronchial veins drain extrapulmonary bronchi, visceral pleura and hilar lymph nodes, end on the right side into the azygos vein and on the left into the left superior intercostal vein or the accessory hemiazygos vein.

(c) False – the left pulmonary artery is higher than the left as it arches over the left main bronchus and descends posterior to it.

(d) True

(e) False – the veins of the upper lobe are anterior to the arteries and bronchi.

13. In the chest:

(a) Air in the oesophagus on axial CT usually indicates a dilated abnormal oesophagus.

(b) On T_2-W MRI the oesophagus shows similar intensity to skeletal muscle.

(c) The thoracic duct transports all of the body lymph into the great veins of the neck.

(d) The thoracic duct is mostly a single structure as it runs from the cisterna chyli.

(e) The thoracic duct crosses from the left to the right at the level of T4.

14. Regarding the mediastinal blood vessels:

(a) The three major aortic branches from right to left are the innominate, left common carotid and left subclavian arteries.

(b) In approximately 0.5% of the population the right subclavian artery arises distal to the left subclavian artery.

(c) The left brachiocephalic vein is anterior to the subclavian, common carotid arteries and trachea.

(d) The internal thoracic veins empty into the corresponding subclavian veins.

(e) The left SVC results from a persistent left cardinal vein.

15. Regarding the mediastinal spaces:

(a) The pretracheal space is bounded anteriorly by the anterior junctional line.

(b) The aortopulmonary window is above the aortic arch.

(c) The aortopulmonary window contains the ligamentum arteriosum and the left recurrent laryngeal nerve.

(d) The azygo-oesophageal recess lies behind the subcarinal space.

(e) The right paratracheal stripe extends down as far as the right tracheobronchial angle.

13.

(a) False – in 80% of normal individuals the oesophagus contains a small amount of air.

(b) False – T_2-W MRI reveals higher intensity than muscle. The signal intensity on T_1-W MRI is similar to that of muscle.

(c) False – all but lymph of most of the lung and the right upper quadrant of the body.

(d) False – it may consist of up to eight separate channels.

(e) False – at T_6, it crosses from right to left of the spine and ascends along the lateral aspect of the oesophagus and arches forward across the left subclavian artery and inserts into a large central vein within 1 cm of the junction of the left internal jugular and subclavian veins.

14.

(a) True

(b) True – the aberrant right subclavian artery runs posterior to the oesophagus from left to right.

(c) True – formed by the junction of left internal and subclavian veins.

(d) False – into the corresponding brachiocephalic veins.

(e) True – in 0.3% to 0.5% of healthy population and in 4.4% to 12.9% of those with congenital heart disease. It usually drains into the coronary sinus, which then communicates with the right atrium.

15.

(a) False – anteriorly the SVC or right brachiocephalic veins, ascending aorta with its enveloping superior pericardial sinus and posteriorly the trachea or carina.

(b) False – above the pulmonary artery under the aortic arch.

(c) True – and fat, though this is not seen on CT due to volume averaging resulting in higher than fat density.

(d) True

(e) True – air containing trachea and lung are separated by a thin layer of fat on the right, giving rise to the 'stripe'. This is broadened at the right tracheobronchial angle by the azygous vein which lies between the airway and the lung.

16. In a chest radiograph:

(a) The anterior junctional line is usually straight and extends to the right ventricle.
(b) The posterior junctional line is anterior to the oesophagus.
(c) The azygo-oesophageal line is below the aortic arch.
(d) The right paravertebral stripe is thicker than that on the left due to the azygos vein.
(e) On a PA projection, the left superior intercostal vein may project lateral to the aortic arch as a small 'nipple'.

17. In the chest:

(a) The thymus is usually inferior to the left brachiocephalic vein.
(b) MRI demonstrates thymic tissue better than CT.
(c) The diaphragmatic crus on the right arises from the upper three lumbar vertebrae.
(d) The oesophageal hiatus lies posterior to the aortic hiatus.
(e) The hiatus for the IVC is posterior to that of the aorta and oesophagus.

18. In the development of the heart:

(a) The primitive heart is formed by fusion of two parallel tubes.
(b) The heart tube kinks to form a U-shaped loop.
(c) The single atrium and ventricle are separated by the dorsal and ventral endocardial cushions.
(d) The foramen secundum is a defect in the septum secundum.
(e) The foramen ovale is due to two overlapping defects, which act like a valve.

16.

(a) True
(b) False – the lungs almost touch each other posterior to the oesophagus to form the posterior junction line.
(c) True – the upper few centimetres are usually straight or concave towards the lung. A convex shape suggests a subcarinal mass in adults; however this may be a normal feature in children.
(d) False – the left paravertebral stripe is usually wider than the right.
(e) True

17.

(a) True – and superior to the level of the horizontal portion of the right pulmonary artery.
(b) True – after puberty, the density gradually decreases owing to fatty replacement. In older patients the thymus may be indistinguishable from mediastinal fat. On T_2-W MRI the signal intensity is similar or sometimes higher than fat and does not change with age. On T_1-W MRI, the intensity of normal thymic tissue is similar or slightly higher than that of muscle.
(c) True – they arch upward and forward to form the margins of the aortic and oesophageal hiati.
(d) False – oesophageal hiatus lies anterior to aortic hiatus.
(e) False – the most anterior of the three diaphragmatic hiati is the hiatus for the IVC, which is in the central tendon immediately beneath the right atrium.

18.

(a) True – soon this grooves to demarcate the sinus venosus, atrium, ventricle and bulbus cordis from behind forward.
(b) True – the caudal end (sinus venosus) receiving venous blood, comes to lie behind the cephalic end (which gives rise to truncus arteriosus). In the fully developed heart, the atria and great vein lie posterior to the ventricles and to the roots of the great arteries.
(c) True – these divide the common atrio-ventricular opening into a right (tricuspid) and left (mitral) orifice.
(d) False – the foramen secundum is a defect in the septum primum.
(e) True – the septum secundum grows to the right of septum primum, is never complete and has a lower free edge. It extends low enough to overlap the foramen secundum and closes it. Ten per cent of individuals have anatomically patent but functionally sealed foramen.

19. In the heart:

(a) The aortic root and pulmonary trunk are covered with parietal pericardium.
(b) The right atrium is anterior and to the right of the left atrium.
(c) The coronary sinus enters the right atrium on the posterior wall.
(d) The crista terminalis demarcates the smooth from the rigid portion of the inner wall of the right atrium.
(e) The Eustachian valve directs blood flow from the IVC into the right atrium in the adult.

20. In the heart:

(a) The pulmonary valve is anterior and to the right of the aortic root.
(b) The interventricular and interatrial septa are in the same plane.
(c) The right ventricle contributes to the right cardiac border on the frontal chest radiograph.
(d) In the right ventricle the crista supraventricularis demarcates the smooth conus from the trabeculated wall.
(e) The moderator band carries the right bundle branch of the conducting system of the right ventricle.

21. Regarding the heart:

(a) The left atrial auricular appendage contributes to the normal left cardiac border.
(b) The left atrium is posterior to the oesophagus.
(c) The four pulmonary veins attach anteriorly in the left atrium.
(d) The left atrium lies to the right of the aortic root.
(e) The mitral valve is placed in the left lower anterior aspect of the left atrium.

22. In the heart:

(a) Most of the external surface of the left ventricle is anterolateral.
(b) The mitral valve lies in the same plane as the tricuspid valve.
(c) The mitral valve is closely related to the non-coronary and left posterior coronary sinuses.

19.

(a) True
(b) True
(c) True
(d) True
(e) False – the Eustachian valve in fetal life serves to direct oxygenated blood from IVC into the foramen ovale. It is rudimentary in adult life.

20.

(a) False – anterior and to the left of the aortic root.
(b) True – left anterior oblique plane.
(c) False – does not usually contribute to the cardiac outline on the frontal chest radiograph.
(d) True
(e) True – crosses from the lower ventricular septum to the anterior papillary muscle.

21.

(a) False – the left atrium does not contribute to the normal cardiac outline.
(b) False – is related posteriorly to the oesophagus and left lower lobe bronchus.
(c) False – the four pulmonary veins are located at the upper and lower margin of the left atrium postero-laterally.
(d) False – it is posterior.
(e) True

22.

(a) False – though the left ventricle forms most of the left heart border on the frontal radiograph, most of its external portion is postero-lateral.
(b) True – right anterior oblique plane.
(c) True – it has no septal attachment.

(d) Each anterior and posterior leaflet of the mitral valve is attached to a papillary muscle by chordae tendinae.

(e) The sinuses of valsalva are below the valve in the aortic root.

23. Regarding the coronary arteries:

(a) Coronary dominance refers to whether the right or left vessels supply the posterior diaphragmatic portion of the interventricular septum and the diaphragmatic surface of the left ventricle.

(b) The right coronary artery runs in the atrioventricular groove.

(c) The posterior descending artery supplies part of the inferior interventricular septum.

(d) The left anterior descending artery runs in the left atrioventricular groove.

(e) In approximately 20% of individuals the LAD tapers before reaching the apex.

24. Regarding the coronary veins:

(a) The anterior cardiac veins empty into the coronary sinus.

(b) The great cardiac vein runs in the anterior interventricular groove.

(c) The middle cardiac vein runs in the left interventricular groove.

(d) Small cardiac veins run with the marginal branches of the right coronary artery.

(e) The left posterior ventricular vein accompanies the posterior descending artery.

25. Regarding the major vessels of the chest:

(a) The aortic arch is anterior to the trachea and oesophagus.

(b) The left pulmonary artery is attached to the junction of the arch and descending aorta.

(c) The left common carotid artery may arise from the brachiocephalic artery.

(d) The aortic hiatus is at the level of T12 vertebra.

(e) The oesophagus is anteromedial to the descending aorta throughout its course.

(d) True
(e) False – the sinuses of valsalva are just above the aortic valve in the aortic root. They are three focal dilatations. The left coronary artery arises from the left posterior sinus, and the right coronary artery arises from the anterior sinus. The right posterior sinus is the non-coronary sinus.

23.

(a) True – 85% of people have right dominance.
(b) True – ultimately anastomosis with the left circumflex artery in the inferior atrioventricular groove.
(c) True
(d) False – the left coronary artery gives off the LAD and the left circumflex artery within one centimetre of its origin. The LAD descends in the anterior interventricular groove.
(e) True – a large septal branch from the LAD may run parallel to the LAD in this case.

24.

(a) False – the anterior cardiac veins drain the anterior surface of the right ventricle and open directly into the right atrium. The venae cordis minimae are minute vessels in the myocardium which also drain into the chambers, mainly the atria.
(b) True – and becomes the coronary sinus.
(c) False – runs in the posterior interventricular groove.
(d) True
(e) False – this vein accompanies the obtuse marginal branches of the left coronary artery.

25.

(a) True
(b) True – the ligamentum arteriosum at the isthmus.
(c) True – commonest variant of the major vessels (27%). The left vertebral may arise directly from the arch (2.5%) and lie between the left common carotid and subclavian arteries.
(d) True
(e) False – in its upper portion the oesophagus lies to the right of the aorta.

26. The superior vena cava:

(a) lies posterior to the right main-stem bronchus.
(b) has direct drainage anteriorly from the azygos vein.
(c) is formed by the union of the right and left brachiocephalic veins.
(d) partly is enclosed in pericardium.
(e) has direct drainage from the internal mammary veins.

27. Regarding the pulmonary artery and vein:

(a) The right main pulmonary artery is beneath the aortic arch.
(b) The right superior pulmonary vein crosses the right main pulmonary artery anteriorly.
(c) The left main pulmonary artery is shorter but in a higher position than that on the right.
(d) The lower lobe pulmonary veins are vertical as they approach the heart.
(e) The pulmonary trunk bifurcates beneath the aortic arch.

26.

(a) False – SVC is anterior to the right main bronchus.
(b) False – the azygos drains into the posterior aspect of the SVC.
(c) True
(d) True
(e) False – the internal mammary veins drain into the corresponding brachiocephalic veins.

27.

(a) True – and in front of the right main bronchus.
(b) True – the hilar point,which is seen on a frontal radiograph. The left is 1 cm higher than that on the right.
(c) True
(d) False – they run horizontally.
(e) True

Limb vasculature and lymphatic system*
A. Doss and M. J. Bull

1. In angiography:

(a) The femoral artery is punctured at its point of minimal pulsation, to prevent haematoma formation.
(b) A low puncture is ideal as it decreases the chances of a retroperitoneal haematoma.
(c) The femoral nerve lies lateral to the artery.
(d) For interventional procedures of the lower limb a retrograde puncture on the ipsilateral femoral artery is ideal.
(e) For punctures of the brachial or axillary arteries, the right arm is usually preferred.

2. In angiography:

(a) The Seldinger technique involves passing a catheter through the puncture needle.
(b) Retrograde popliteal artery puncture is useful for angioplasty of the superficial femoral artery.
(c) Intravenous digital subtraction angiography usually requires less iodinated contrast medium than the intra-arterial technique.
(d) Radial artery catheterization is performed using a 5F catheter.
(e) Translumbar approach to the aorta is the best way of visualizing the aorta.

3. In the upper chest:

(a) The right subclavian artery arises directly from the arch of the aorta.
(b) The subclavian artery lies posterior to the subclavian vein.

---

* From *Applied Radiological Anatomy:* 'The limb vasculature and the lymphatic system'.

Limb vasculature and lymphatic system*
ANSWERS

1.

(a) False – point of maximal pulsation usually as it passes over the medial third of the femoral head.

(b) False – a high puncture placed above the inguinal ligament may result in retroperitoneal haematoma as the artery is difficult to compress without the support of the femoral head. A low puncture may cause a pseudoaneurysm formation or arteriovenous fistula if the profunda femoris is punctured.

(c) True – so a large haematoma may compress and damage the nerve.

(d) False – an antegrade puncture, so that catheters and wires can be passed down the leg easily.

(e) False – the left arm, avoids manipulation of catheters across origin of great vessels.

2.

(a) False – a guide wire is passed through the needle into the artery. The needle is removed and a catheter is passed over the guide wire into the artery.

(b) True

(c) False – requires large amounts.

(d) False – 3F catheters usually.

(e) False – largely abandoned nowadays, and replaced by the aortogram through the transfemoral approach.

3.

(a) False – usually from the brachiocephalic trunk which divides into the right subclavian and right common carotid arteries. The left subclavian arises directly from the arch of the aorta.

(b) True – and scalenus anterior muscle and ends at the lateral border of the first rib, where it continues as the axillary artery.

* From *Applied Radiological Anatomy:* 'The limb vasculature and the lymphatic system'.

(c) The dorsal scapular artery arises from the second part of the subclavian artery.
(d) The suprascapular artery arises from the thyro-cervical trunk.
(e) The inferior thyroid artery contributes to the blood supply of the spinal cord.

4. Regarding the axillary artery:

(a) The subclavian artery continues as the axillary artery at the lateral border of teres major muscle.
(b) The pectoralis major muscle divides the axillary artery into three parts.
(c) The cords of the brachial plexus are anterior to the second part of the axillary artery.
(d) The subscapular artery runs downwards on the posterior axillary wall to the inferior angle of the scapula.
(e) The third part is superficial and may be used for arterial puncture.

5. Regarding the arteries of the forearm and hand:

(a) The brachial artery divides into radial and ulnar arteries at the level of the neck of the radius.
(b) The profunda brachi artery runs in the radial groove.
(c) The brachial artery is superficial to the bicipital aponeurosis.
(d) The radial artery may branch off higher than the usual level.
(e) The radial artery gives off the common interosseus artery 2 cm below its origin.

6. In the lower abdomen and pelvis:

(a) There are no terminal branches to the aorta.
(b) The common iliac arteries divide at the level of the sacroiliac joints.
(c) The common iliac arteries lie in front of the fourth and fifth lumbar vertebrae.
(d) The ureters lie anterior to the common iliac arteries.
(e) The superior rectal artery lies anterior to the right common iliac artery.

(c)   True – and supplies muscles attached to the medial border of the scapula and takes part in the scapular anastomosis with the third part of the axillary artery.

(d)   True – and so do inferior thyroid and superficial cervical artery.

(e)   True – and so does the ascending cervical artery.

4.

(a)   False – lateral border of first rib to the lower border of teres major muscle is the axillary artery, after which it is the brachial artery.

(b)   False – pectoralis minor divides it into three parts.

(c)   False – they surround this artery medially, laterally and posteriorly and separate it from the axillary vein which runs medially and slightly anteriorly.

(d)   True – and contributes to the scapular anastomosis.

(e)   True

5.

(a)   True

(b)   True – gives branches to scapular and elbow anastomosis.

(c)   False – superficial throughout its course and overlapped by bicipital aponeurosis at the elbow.

(d)   True – 'high take-off' of radial artery – a common normal variant above the neck of the radius. The deep palmar arch is a continuation of the radial artery.

(e)   False – ulnar artery.

6.

(a)   False – three; a pair of common iliac arteries and the median sacral artery anterior and to the left of the body of L4 vertebra.

(b)   True – into the internal and external iliac arteries.

(c)   True

(d)   True – common iliac veins, lumbosacral trunk, obturator nerve, iliolumbar artery and the sympathetic trunk lie posterior to the common iliac trunk.

(e)   False – anterior to the left common iliac artery.

7. In the pelvis and lower abdomen:

(a) The superior gluteal artery is a branch of the external iliac artery.

(b) The uterine artery is a branch of the anterior division of the internal iliac artery.

(c) The umbilical artery is the first branch of the internal iliac artery in the fetus.

(d) The internal pudendal artery re-enters the pelvis through the lesser sciatic foramen.

(e) The inferior epigastric artery is given off above the inguinal ligament from the external iliac artery.

8. In the lower limb:

(a) The main supply to the trochanteric anastomosis is through the superficial femoral artery.

(b) The superficial femoral artery passes lateral to and behind the lower shaft of the femur.

(c) The popliteal artery lies lateral to the popliteal vein in the popliteal fossa.

(d) The descending genicular artery is a branch of the popliteal artery supplying the knee.

(e) The anterior tibial artery runs anterior to the interosseous membrane.

9. Regarding the veins of the lower limbs and abdomen:

(a) Failure of the right subcardinal vein to connect with the liver leads to absence of the IVC.

(b) A persistent left sacrocardinal vein results in a left-sided IVC.

(c) The right common iliac vein is crossed by the common iliac artery.

(d) The hepatic segment of the IVC is formed from the right vitelline vein.

(e) A left-sided IVC drains into the coronary sinus.

10. In the lymphatic system:

(a) Lipiodol is retained in lymph nodes for about 12 months.

(b) The upper limit of normal in the short axis for retrocrural nodes is 10 mm.

7.

(a) False – largest branch of the posterior division of the internal iliac artery, passes through greater sciatic foramen.
(b) True – runs in the broad ligament.
(c) True – persists as the fibrous medial umbilical ligament, which may be recognized in a plain abdominal film in the presence of a pneumoperitoneum.
(d) True – supplies the genitalia.
(e) True – runs up on the deep surface of the anterior abdominal wall and enters the rectus sheath.

8.

(a) False – this anastomosis supplies the femoral head and is formed by anastomosing branches of lateral and medial circumflex femoral and superior gluteal arteries.
(b) False – posterior and medial to the femur, through the adductor hiatus.
(c) False – this artery lies deep to the popliteal vein.
(d) False – this is a branch of the superficial femoral artery, prior to entering the adductor hiatus. The medial and lateral superior and inferior genicular arteries are given off in the popliteal fossa.
(e) True – in the lower leg, the artery passes deep to the extensor retinaculum, and can be palpated lateral to the extensor hallucis longus tendon and continues as the dorsalis pedis artery.

9.

(a) True – the drainage of the lower body is through the azygos system and SVC. Absent IVC is associated with cardiac abnormalities.
(b) True
(c) False – this is true with that of the left.
(d) True – the other segments are renal and sacrocardinal.
(e) False – due to a persistent left sacrocardinal vein, cross-over to the right IVC occurs at the level of the left renal vein.

10.

(a) True – used to monitor nodal size following therapy.
(b) False – 6 mm, para-aortic and subcarinal nodes may be up to 12 mm.

(c) Fifty per cent of patients demonstrate cross-drainage of lymphatics from right to left at the level of L3/4.
(d) The cisterna chyli continues upwards through the aortic opening in the diaphragm as the thoracic duct.
(e) The thoracic duct drains the whole of the chest and limbs.

(c) True – lumbar gap – non-opacification of nodes at this level on lymphography.
(d) True
(e) False – the thoracic duct drains all the body below the diaphragm, posterior right chest wall and left of the body above the diaphragm. The right lymph duct drains the remainder.

Module 2

Musculoskeletal and soft tissue (including trauma)

A. Doss and M. J. Bull

1. The following are true:

(a) The supraspinatus tendon passes above the acromion process.
(b) The clavicle has a medullary cavity.
(c) The rhomboid fossa marks the site of origin of the costo-clavicular ligament.
(d) The clavicle is the last bone to ossify.
(e) A distance of less than 5 mm between the humerus and the acromion indicates likely supraspinatus tendon impingement.

2. Regarding the shoulder joint:

(a) The capsule of the shoulder joint is lax inferiorly.
(b) The long head of the biceps runs under the transverse humeral ligament.
(c) The subscapularis bursa is a herniation of the shoulder joint synovial membrane deep to the subscapularis muscle, through a defect in the glenohumeral ligament.
(d) Teres major forms part of the rotator cuff.
(e) During shoulder arthrography contrast passes normally into the subacromial bursa.

3. Regarding the shoulder joint:

(a) CT arthrography is of value in the assessment of the glenoid labrum.
(b) T_2-W images and STIR (short tau inversion recovery) sequences with fat suppression can identify tears in the supraspinatus tendon.
(c) On ultrasound, the supraspinatus tendon is echobright.
(d) In anterior dislocation of the shoulder, cortical defects may occur in the anterior aspect of the head of the humerus.

Musculoskeletal and soft tissue (including trauma)
ANSWERS

1.

(a) False – below the acromion.
(b) False – there is no medullary cavity because of its mesenchymal origin.
(c) True – in 5% of individuals an irregular groove is in the inferomedial aspect of the clavicle from which the costoclavicular ligament arises to insert into the first costal cartilage.
(d) False – first bone to ossify, formed in membrane, appears after the first fetal month.
(e) True

2.

(a) True – attached proximally to the glenoid labrum and distally to the anatomical neck of the humerus.
(b) True
(c) True
(d) False – teres minor, subscapularis, supraspinatus, infraspinatus – prime function of these muscle is to hold the head of the humerus in the glenoid cavity during all movement.
(e) False – contrast or air in the subacromial space implies disruption of the supra spinatus tendon.

3.

(a) True – the prone oblique position provides more information about the posterior aspect of the glenoid labrum and the capsular attachments, which are important in patients with posterior dislocations.
(b) True – the supraspinatus tendon is best seen in the coronal oblique plane.
(c) False – the tendinous margin is echobright and central portion is echopoor.
(d) False – they occur in the posterior aspect of the head of the humerus (Hill–Sachs lesion), which are best shown by a Striker's view (patient supine, humerus 90° to the table with a cephald beam at 25°).

(e) All the rotator cuff muscles are attached to the greater tubercle of the humerus.

4. Regarding the upper limb:

(a) The radial groove is situated in the radius.
(b) The capitulum articulates with the ulna.
(c) The ligament of Struthers may compress the median nerve.
(d) The capitulum is the first secondary ossification centre to appear in the elbow.
(e) A prominent posterior fat pad in a lateral radiograph of the elbow is seen in cases of joint effusion.

5. In the upper limb:

(a) The annular ligament of the elbow blends with the ulnar collateral ligament.
(b) The bicipital aponeurosis separates the superficial median cubital vein from the deeper brachial artery.
(c) The ulna articulates with the carpal bones.
(d) The distal radio-ulnar joint has no communication with the carpal joints.
(e) The ulna articulates with the triquetral only during ulnar deviation of the wrist.

6. Concerning the wrist and carpus:

(a) The mid-carpal joint does not communicate with the radiocarpal joint.
(b) On a lateral wrist radiograph the distal radius has a slight volar tilt.
(c) The lunate articulates proximally with the radius and distally with the capitate.
(d) The flexor retinaculum is attached to the pisiform, hook of hamate, scaphoid tubercle and ridge of the trapezium.
(e) Flexor carpi-radialis attaches to the pisiform.

(e) False – all but the subscapularis, which is attached to the lesser tubercle of the humerus.

4.

(a) False – within the radial groove runs the radial nerve and the profunda brachialis artery. This groove is closely applied to the mid shaft of the humerus and a fracture in this location may give rise to neuropraxia.

(b) False – capitulum–radial head; trochea – ulna.

(c) True – this ligament runs from a supracondylar spur (which may be seen in less than 1% of individuals) to the medial epicondyle with the median nerve and brachial artery beneath it.

(d) True – the order in which they appear are as follows: capitulum (1 year), radial head and medial (internal) epicondyle (5 years), trochlea (11 years), olecranon (12 years), lateral (external) epicondyle (13 years) – use the mnemonic CRITOE.

(e) True – a prominent anterior fat pad is a normal variant in 15% of individuals.

5.

(a) False – it blends with the radial collateral ligament, surrounds the head of the radius like a horseshoe and is attached to the ulna medially.

(b) True

(c) False – the radius carries the hand. The lower extremity of the radius expands to form the articular surface for the wrist joint and the ulna.

(d) True – if a communication is demonstrated at arthrography, the triangular fibrocartilage must be disrupted.

(e) False

6.

(a) True

(b) True – if this is lost, a fracture of the radius should be suspected.

(c) True

(d) True – this forms the carpal tunnel which contains tendons of flexor pollicis longus, flexor digitorum profundus and superficialis and the median nerve. The tendon of flexor carpiradialis lies in a separate compartment of the carpal tunnel

(e) False – flexor carpi-ulnaris.

7. In the hand and wrist:

(a) In most cases two views are enough to exclude scaphoid fractures.
(b) In 15% of cases blood supply is from the distal to the proximal portion of the scaphoid.
(c) The scaphoid ossifies in the sixth year.
(d) All the metacarpals articulate with each other and with the corresponding carpal bones.
(e) The commonest supernumerary bone of the wrist joint is the os radiale.

8. In skeletal imaging:

(a) Phased array surface detection coils greatly improve the signal to noise ratio in MRI of bone joint and soft tissue.
(b) Abnormalities of cortical bone and calcification are usually not detected by MRI.
(c) Meniscal abnormalities of the knee are best demonstrated on T_1-weighted scans.
(d) A fat fluid level within the suprapatellar bursa of the knee joint indicates a fracture within the joint.
(e) Bone scans using 99mTc MDP are very specific for pathology.

9. In the bony pelvis:

(a) the triradiate cartilage is seen as a Y-shaped lucency at the acetabulum in an immature skeleton in a plain radiograph.
(b) the iliac crest has a separate ossification centre.
(c) the rectus femoris originates at the anterior superior iliac spine.
(d) the obturator foramen is bounded inferiorly by the sacro-spinous ligaments.
(e) the sacrotuberous ligament defines the posterior limit of the lesser sciatic foramen.

7.

(a) False – four views are necessary, as fractures are easily missed – antero-posterior, 30° antero-posterior, lateral and scaphoid centred view.
(b) True – hence fractures at the waist may produce ischaemic necrosis of the proximal portion.
(c) True – so do trapezium and trapezoid. Capitate and hamate ossify in the first year, triquetral in the second, lunate in the third, pisiform in the twelfth year.
(d) False – all but the first metacarpals which articulate only with the trapezium.
(e) True – lies immediately distal to the radial styloid.

8.

(a) True
(b) True
(c) False – T_2 Fast spin echo sequence.
(d) True – lipohaemarthrosis seen in a lateral radiograph of the knee.
(e) False – a three-phase study is used – immediate vascular images (0.3 minutes), a blood-pool phase (3–5 minutes), and delayed static images (4–6 hours). Bone scan is very sensitive to the presence of any pathology, but is relatively non-specific. Hot spots are due to increased blood supply or osteoblast activity and may be seen in infection, fracture or malignancy.

9.

(a) True – the ilium, ischium and pubis meet at the triradiate cartilage, fuses at 20 years of age.
(b) True – fuses from 20 years onwards.
(c) False – Sartorius originates at the anterior Superior iliac spine and rectus femoris from the anterior inferior iliac spine. It is common for 'tug' lesions (avulsion) to develop from the latter in sports related injuries of adolescents.
(d) False – the obturator foramen is bounded by the bodies and rami of the pubis and ischium. The sacrospinous ligament defines the inferior limit of the greater sciatic foramen.
(e) True – runs from the ischial tuberosity to the side of the sacrum and coccyx and to the posterior inferior iliac spine.

10. In the pelvis:

(a) The iliopsoas muscle passes anterior to the inguinal ligament.
(b) The aponeurosis of the external oblique has a thickening, which runs from the pubic tubercle to the anterior superior iliac spine as the inguinal ligament.
(c) The sacroiliac joint does not have a synovial component.
(d) The intersosseous sacroiliac ligament is a strong ligament.
(e) Each half of the vertebral arch of the sacrum appears at 16–20 weeks of fetal life.

11. Concerning the muscles of the pelvic girdle:

(a) The majority of the gluteus maximus merges with the iliotibial tract.
(b) The piriformis passes out of the pelvis through the lesser sciatic foramen.
(c) The obturator internus arises from the medial part of the obturator membrane and surrounding bone and passes through the lesser sciatic foramen.
(d) The gemelli muscles insert into the lesser trochanter.
(e) The tendons of obturator internus and gemelli muscles lie between the femoral head anteriorly and gluteus maximus posteriorly.

12. In the pelvis:

(a) The anteroposterior view of the plain radiograph is taken with the legs rotated externally.
(b) The paraglenoid sulcus transmits the superior branch of the gluteal artery.
(c) Shenton's line runs from the lateral aspect of the femoral neck to the superior border of the obturator foramen on an AP radiograph.
(d) The sacrum is better seen with a 35° cephalad angulation on the AP radiograph.
(e) The sacroiliac joints are better profiled in the postero-anterior than the anteroposterior projection.

10.

(a) False – posterior, to insert into the lesser trochanter.
(b) True
(c) False – has a synovial component. The sacral surface is lined by fibrocartilage and the iliac surface by hyaline cartilage.
(d) True – it provides the main strength of the joint.
(e) True

11.

(a) True
(b) False – through the greater sciatic foramen.
(c) True
(d) False – the gemellus inferior arises from the ischial tuberosity and the gemellus superior arises from the ischial spine and insert into the greater trochanter.
(e) True

12.

(a) False – rotated internally to compensate for the anteversion of the femoral neck.
(b) True
(c) False – from the medial aspect of the femoral neck it usually is a smooth curve.
(d) True – Ferguson's view. The Stork's view to assess instability of the pubic symphysis is taken standing on each leg. Change in alignment of the superior surface of the pubic rami of more than 3 mm is abnormal.
(e) True – the plane of the SI joint diverges in the posteroanterior direction and the diverging X-ray beam is nearly parallel in the PA view.

13. In pelvimetry:

(a) Routine assessment of the female pelvis is performed before delivery.
(b) CT or MRI are used in place of plain radiography.
(c) The conjugate diameter is the smallest AP diameter between the posterior margin of the symphysis pubis and the anterior aspect of the sacrum.
(d) The pelvic outlet dimensions are more important than the inlet dimensions.
(e) The transverse outlet diameter is measured between the ischial tuberosities.

14. In the hip joint:

(a) The fovea capitis to which the ligamentum teres is attached is not covered in cartilage.
(b) The articular cartilage is thickest and broadest superiorly.
(c) The fibrous capsule is attached around the rim of the acetabulum and inferiorly to the transverse acetabular ligament.
(d) The iliofemoral ligament is a thickening of the posterior capsule.
(e) The Von Rosen's view is useful in the assessment of femoral capital epiphyses in children.

15. Regarding the femur:

(a) MRI has a high sensitivity and specificity in detecting avascular necrosis of the femoral head.
(b) The anteversion of the neck of the femur increases from childhood into adult life.
(c) The principal blood supply to the head of the adult femur is from the medial and lateral circumflex femoral arteries.
(d) The nutrient artery of the femur travels cranially.
(e) The medial condyle is smaller than the lateral condyle.

13.

(a) False
(b) True
(c) True – the most important measurement. Normal range is 11–12.5 cm.Less than 10.5 cm indicates increasing likelihood of cephalopelvic disproportion.
(d) False – there is a considerable increase in the outlet diameter of up to 4 cm during delivery due to relaxation of the symphysis pubis and rotation of the sacroiliac joints.
(e) True – average is 10.5 cm.

14.

(a) True
(b) True
(c) True – where the weight is borne.
(d) False – this is the ischio-femoral ligament. The ilio-femoral ligament is attached to the anterior inferior iliac spine and to the inter-rochanteric line, and is anterior to the femoral neck.
(e) False – the Frog's lateral view is used for this – the Von Rosen's view is used in the assessment of congenital dislocation of the hip. Judet's views of the acetabulum and femoral head give information on the anterior and posterior columns of the acetabulum.

15.

(a) True
(b) False – in children the anteversion is greater, 50° at 1 year, 25° at 3–5 years and 8° by adulthood.
(c) True – the central part of the head may be supplied by the artery of ligamentum teres, a branch of the obturator artery. This may be absent in about 20% of individuals. Intracapsular fractures of the femoral neck can compromise the blood supply to the head of the femur as the circumflex arteries may be torn. This gives rise to a high incidence of avascular necrosis of the femoral head or non-union.
(d) True – 'Flee from the knee'. On a lateral view this is not to be mistaken for a fracture.
(e) False – larger. Hence the inferior surface of the femur is nearly horizontal despite the shaft being oblique.

16. In the lower limb:

(a) The patella is a sesamoid bone within the quadriceps tendon.
(b) The fabella is frequently found in the lateral head of gastrocnemius.
(c) The shaft of the femur ossifies at the 35th week of fetal life.
(d) In a bipartite patella the supero-lateral part is separate to the rest of the patella.
(e) Tensor fascia lata arises from the anterior superior iliac spine and inserts into the lateral condyle of the femur.

17. In the lower limb:

(a) The rectus femoris arises from the anterior superior iliac spine.
(b) Gracilis, sartorius and semitendinosus insert into the medial condyle of the tibia.
(c) The adductor magnus inserts along the linea aspera, the medial supracondylar line and the adductor tubercle of the medial femoral condyle.
(d) The adductor hiatus interrupts the distal attachment of the adductor longus muscle.
(e) The biceps femoris attaches to the lateral condyle of the femur.

18. In the knee joint:

(a) The synovium lining the joint is extracapsular.
(b) A Baker's cyst is an inflamed or swollen medial gastrocnemius – semimembranosus bursa.
(c) The lateral collateral ligament is separated from the capsule by the popliteus tendon.
(d) The anterior cruciate ligament passes from the anterior intercondylar area of the tibia to the medial femoral condyle.
(e) The medial collateral ligament is a flattened band that blends posteriorly with the fibrous capsule.

16.

(a) True – largest sesamoid bone.
(b) True – a fabeLLa – 'L' for lateral.
(c) False – starts to ossify at the seventh week of fetal life.
(d) True – usually bilateral. May be difficult to differentiate from a fracture.
(e) False – inserts into the iliotibial tract – a strong thickened band of deep fascia of the lateral aspect of the thigh (fascia lata) which is attached to the lateral condyle of the tibia.

17.

(a) False – from the anterior inferior iliac spine. The sartorius and tensor fascia lata arise from the anterior superior iliac spine. The rectus femoris inserts into the base of the patella and by the patellar ligament to the tibial tuberosity. This insertion is the same for the other muscles which form the quadriceps femoris; vastus – lateralis, medialis and intermedius.
(b) True
(c) True
(d) False – the femoral vessels pass through the hiatus in the adductor magnus to become the popliteal vessels.
(e) False – originates from the ischial tuberosity (long head) and the linea aspera (short head) and inserts into the head of the fibula.

18.

(a) False – intracapsular.
(b) True – best seen on ultrasound as an anechoic area that may connect to the knee joint.
(c) True – it is a cord-like structure between the lateral epicondyle of the femur and head of the fibula.
(d) False – to the medial surface of lateral femoral condyle. It prevents femur moving backwards on tibia.
(e) True

19. In the knee joint:

(a) The anterior cruciate ligament has low signal intensity on T_1- and T_2-weighted sagittal scans.
(b) The posterior cruciate ligament (PCL) arises from the posterior intercondylar area and inserts into the anterior part of the lateral surface of the medial femoral condyle.
(c) The medial meniscus is larger and more semicircular than the lateral meniscus.
(d) Discoid menisci are less likely to tear than normal menisci.
(e) The posterior horn of the lateral meniscus is attached to medial condyle of the femur by the menisco-femoral ligament, which divides to pass either side of the anterior cruciate ligament.

20. In the knee:

(a) A tunnel view shows the patella well.
(b) The medial femoral condyle projects more anteriorly compared to the lateral femoral condyle.
(c) A fat fluid level in the suprapatellar bursa in a horizontal beam lateral radiograph indicates a fracture within the joint.
(d) The sartorius and gracilis tendons are posteromedial to the joint.
(e) The popliteal vein lies deep to the popliteal artery.

21. Regarding the lower legs:

(a) The muscles of the anterior compartment are more prone to be affected by compartmental syndrome.

19.

(a) True – partial tear may manifest as high signal within the ligament on T_2 or $T_2{}^*$ images. More often a torn ACL is not visualized. Coronal images show medial and lateral collateral ligaments, sagittal images show menisci, cruciate ligaments and articular cartilages. Normal menisci and ligaments are low signal on T_1 and T_2.

(b) True – the PCL is shorter and stronger than the ACL. It is infrequently torn compared with ACL.

(c) True – the outer margin of the medial meniscus is blended with the fibrous capsule and the deep surface of the medial collateral ligament.

(d) False – discoid menisci are thicker. However, more prone to tear and may be symptomatic even if not torn.

(e) False – pass either side of PCL. The anterior part is called ligament of Humphrey and the posterior part, ligament of Wrisberg. One or the other can be seen in about 70% of cases. They can be mistaken for a tear of the posterior horn of the lateral meniscus or for loose bodies in front of or behind the PCL.

20.

(a) False – a skyline view of the patella shows it best. A tunnel view of the intercondylar fossa of the upper end of the tibia is used to detect intra-articular opacities. These opacities are 'loose' bodies if they change position.

(b) False – the lateral femoral condyle projects more anteriorly and tends to prevent lateral dislocation.

(c) True – has a high correlation with a tibial plateau fracture – probably the most commonly missed fracture of the knee.

(d) True

(e) False – the vein is superficial to the artery. Hence during Doppler ultrasound for venous thrombosis, excess pressure with the probe will obliterate the lumen and it cannot be visualized. This applies to ultrasound of veins in general. However, this is a sign to be elicited with the probe held transverse to the vein, to ensure patency of veins.

21.

(a) True – they are in a compartment enclosed by the tibia, fibula and the interosseus membrane.

(b) The Achilles tendon has a sheath.
(c) The tibialis anterior is the most medial and the largest of the flexor tendons of the foot.
(d) The flexor digitorum longus tendon is lateral to flexor hallucis longus at the level of the talus.
(e) The tibialis posterior inserts into the talus.

22. In the ankle and the foot:

(a) The deltoid ligament lies medially, deep to the flexor tendons.
(b) The deltoid ligament is responsible for about 85% of all ankle ligament injuries.
(c) The tibiofibular and calcaneofibular ligaments form the superior group of the lateral collateral ligament complex in the ankle.
(d) The sinus tarsus is a space between the talus and calcaneus and is filled with fat and hindfoot ligaments.
(e) Tarsal coalition is usually of no consequence.

23. Concerning imaging of the ankle and foot:

(a) Boehler's angle is usually about 28°.
(b) Congenital tarsal coalitions are best visualized using oblique radiographs with the foot internally rotated.
(c) On ultrasound, tendons are echopoor.
(d) In the AP view of the foot the medial margin of the base of the second metatarsal should be in line with the medial margin of the intermediate cuneiform.
(e) A fracture through the base of the fifth metatarsal is usually longitudinal to the long axis of the metatarsal.

(b) False – strongest tendon, but no sheath, therefore tenosynovitis does not accur.
(c) False – this is the tibialis posterior which provides support to the longitudinal arch. Problems in the arch can lead to tendonitis or even rupture usually just at or above the tibiotalar joint.
(d) False – the mnemonic **T**om (**t**ibialis posterior), **D**ick (flexor **d**igitorum longus), **a**nd (posterior tibial vessels **a**nd nerve), **H**arry (flexor **h**allucis longus) is helpful in remembering the relations of these important structures at the level of the ankle joint from medial to the poserto-lateral aspect.
(e) False – talus has no muscle attachment. The tibialis posterior inserts into the navicular, and gives variable slips to tarsal bodies and bases of second, third and fourth metatarsals.

22.

(a) True
(b) False – the lateral collateral ligament complex is responsible for about 80% of all ankle ligament injuries.
(c) False – these form the inferior group. The superior group is formed by the anterior and posterior tibial and fibular ligaments. The anterior talofibular ligament is the most commonly torn ligament in the ankle.
(d) True – in the sinus tarsi syndrome this fat is obliterated with disruption of the ligaments.
(e) False – this is a common cause of a painful flat foot. The coalition which may be bony, cartilagenous or fibrous, most commonly occurs at the calcaneo-navicular joint and is usually bilateral.

23.

(a) True – an angle less than 20° indicates flattening of the calcaneum due to crush injuries resulting from jumping on to a hard surface from a height.
(b) False – CT, particularly in the coronal plane, is the best way of looking at the subtalar joint.
(c) False – tendons are echobright. Echopoor areas in the tendon may be due to tendonitis and a gap in the tendon is diagnostic of a tear.
(d) True – in the oblique view of the foot, the medial margin of the base of the third metatarsal should be in line with the medial margin of the lateral cuneiform. If not, it is a Lisfranc injury.
(e) False – avulsion fracture of the base of the fifth metatarsal is transverse to the long axis of the metatarsal. An apophysis which mimics a fracture is longitudinal to the long axis of the metatarsal.

Module 3

Gastro-intestinal (including hepatobiliary)

A. Doss and M. J. Bull

1. Regarding the abdomen:

(a) By the fifth week of fetal life the gut tube within the peritoneal cavity is suspended by the dorsal mesentery.
(b) The blind ending hind gut is closed by the cloacal membrane.
(c) The superior mesenteric artery supplies the gut from the inferior half of the duodenum to the splenic flexure.
(d) The coeliac axis supplies the gut from the upper oeosphagus to the superior half of the duodenum.
(e) The inferior mesenteric artery supplies the hind gut distal to the hepatic flexure up to the anal canal.

2. During embryological development:

(a) A condensation of endoderm in the dorsal mesogastrium forms the spleen.
(b) In the third week of fetal life the liver arises from a hepatic diverticulum which buds from the duodenum.
(c) The dorsal pancreatic bud arises from the hepatic diverticulum.
(d) The pancreas may form a complete ring around the duodenum.
(e) The ventral pancreatic duct forms the accessory pancreatic duct.

3. In the development of the gut:

(a) The cranial limb of the primary intestinal loop gives rise to most of the ileum.
(b) During the sixth week of fetal life the midgut herniates into the umbilical cord.

Gastro-intestinal (including hepatobiliary)
ANSWERS

1.

(a) True
(b) True
(c) True
(d) False – from the lower oesophagus.
(e) False – distal to the splenic flexure up to the upper half of the anal canal.

2.

(a) False – the spleen develops as a condensation of mesenchyme in the dorsal mesogastrium of the lesser sac during the fifth week. It is derived from mesoderm and not from gut endoderm.
(b) True – the gall bladder and cystic duct develop from a further budding from the hepatic diverticulum.
(c) False – the dorsal bud develops from the duodenum opposite the hepatic diverticulum from which sprouts the ventral diverticulum. The dorsal bud gives rise to the head, body and tail of the pancreas. The ventral bud develops into the uncinate process.
(d) True – annular pancreas probably results from a bilobed ventral bud with the two lobes migrating in opposite directions, around the duodenum to fuse with the dorsal bud.
(e) False – the ventral pancreatic duct becomes the main pancreatic duct of Wirsung. The dorsal pancreatic duct forms the accessory duct of Santorini.

3.

(a) True – the caudal limb develops into the ascending and transverse colon.
(b) True – as it herniates into the umbilicus the primary intestinal loop rotates around the axis of the superior mesenteric vessels through 90° in an anti-clockwise direction.

(c) During the 24th week of fetal life the midgut retracts into the abdomen.
(d) The mesenteries of the ascending and descending colon blend with the posterior peritoneal wall.
(e) The lower part of the anal canal is ectodermal in origin.

4. In developmental anomalies of the gut:

(a) Failure of recanalization of the lumen of the midgut may result in atresia or stenosis of the bowel.
(b) Meckel's diverticulum represents the remains of the embryonic right umbilical vein.
(c) In an undescended caecum, neonatal intestinal obstruction is caused by Ladd's band.
(d) Ischaemic changes to the bowel in the fetal umbilical hernia may result in atresia or stenosis of the bowel.
(e) The embryonic vitello intestinal duct gives rise to the appendix.

5. Regarding the peritoneum:

(a) It is a closed sac in both male and female.
(b) The greater and lesser sac communicate through the epiploic foramen.
(c) The flow of peritoneal fluid is directed in a cephalad direction by the negative intra-abdominal pressure generated in the upper abdomen by respiration.
(d) The peritoneal cavity is divided by the greater omentum into the supramesocolic and inframesocolic compartments.
(e) The root of the transverse mesocolon extends from the infra-ampullary segment of the duodenum through the head and along the lower edge of the body and tail of the pancreas.

6. Concerning the peritoneal spaces:

(a) The right subphrenic space extends from the right coronary ligament postero-inferiorly to the falciform ligament medially.
(b) In the supine position the hepatorenal space (Morrison's pouch) is more dependant than the right paracolic gutter.
(c) The lesser sac is posterior to the pancreas.
(d) Fluid collections in the pelvis that spread to the left subphrenic space, generally involve the lesser sac.

(c) False – in the tenth week it rotates counter-clockwise through 180° and the cephalic limb returns first, passing upwards into the space in the left of the abdomen.

(d) True – this forms an avascular plane, which the surgeon employs to mobilize the right and left colon.

(e) True – an ectodermal invagination termed proctodeum. The pectinate line in the adult marks the junction of the ectoderm and endoderm in the anal canal.

4.

(a) True – in the sixth week of fetal life, proliferation of the endodermal lining of the gut completely occludes its lumen. Recanalization takes place and is completed by the ninth week. Incomplete recanalization may lead to gut duplication.

(b) False

(c) True – the peritoneal fold which normally seals the caecum in the right iliac fossa passes across the duodenum (Ladd 's band) and causes a neonatal intestinal obstruction. The small bowel mesentery in this case is a narrow pedicle and allows volvulus of the whole small intestine – volvulus neonatorum.

(d) True

(e) False – it may persist as Meckel's diverticulum.

5.

(a) False – closed in the male, penetrated by the fallopian tubes in the female.

(b) True – foramen of Winslow.

(c) True – and is directed by gravity.

(d) False – the transverse mesocolon and transverse colon divide the peritoneal cavity.

(e) True

6.

(a) True – the falci form ligament separates it from the left subphrenic space.

(b) True – hence a common site for collections.

(c) False – anterior to pancreas, behind and to the left of the stomach.

(d) False – the splenorenal and gastrosplenic ligaments limit the lesser sac on the left. Therefore fluid collection spreading into the left subphrenic space does not involve the lesser sac.

(e) Subphrenic collections are more common on the left than the right.

7. Concerning the peritoneal spaces:

(a) The right inframesocolic space is in direct communication with the pelvis.
(b) The paracolic gutters are retroperitoneal recesses on the posterior abdominal wall lateral to the ascending and descending colon.
(c) There are two potential spaces posterior to the bladder in women.
(d) In the supine position the Pouch of Douglas is the most dependent portion of the peritoneum.
(e) The peritoneum is reflected on the prostate.

8. In the pelvic peritoneum:

(a) The rectum is covered by peritoneum on the front up to the junction of the middle and lower thirds.
(b) The peritoneum is reflected on the infero-lateral aspect of the bladder bilaterally.
(c) The broad ligaments contain the fallopian tubes.
(d) The left limb of the sigmoid mesocolon is attached medially to the left psoas muscle.
(e) The left ureter runs in the apex of the sigmoid mesocolon.

9. In the abdomen:

(a) The superior mesenteric vessels lie in the small bowel mesentery.
(b) The root of the transverse mesocolon is confluent with the root of the small bowel mesentery.
(c) The greater omentum inserts into the antero-superior aspect of the transverse colon.

(e) False – the phrenicocolic ligament extends from the splenic flexure of the colon
     to the diaphragm, partially separates the left posterior subphrenic space from
     the rest of the peritoneal cavity. It forms a partial barrier to the spread of fluid
     from the left paracolic gutter into the left subphrenic space which is why right-
     sided collections are more common than left-sided collections.

7.

(a) False – the inframesocolic compartment is divided into the smaller right and
     larger left spaces by the root of the small bowel mesentery which runs from the
     duodenojejunal flexure to the ileocaecal valve. The right inframesocolic
     compartment is bounded by the transverse colon and the root of the small
     bowel mesentery. The left inframesocolic space is in free communication with
     the pelvis on the right of the midline and the mesentery of the sigmoid colon
     forms a partial barrier on the left of the midline.
(b) False – these are peritoneal recesses. Both are in continuity with the pelvic
     peritoneal spaces.
(c) True – the rectouterine pouch of Douglas and the utero-vesical pouch. Men
     have one potential space posterior to the bladder – the recto-vesical pouch.
(d) True
(e) False

8.

(a) True
(b) False – it is reflected over the fundus of the bladder.
(c) True – the layers of peritoneum on the anterior and posterior surfaces of the
     uterus are reflected laterally as the broad ligaments.
(d) True
(e) False – the sigmoid and superior rectal vessels run between the layers of the
     sigmoid mesocolon and the left ureter runs behind its apex into the pelvis.

9.

(a) True – in front of the horizontal part of the duodenum.
(b) True – near the uncinate process of the pancreas. The middle colic vessels
     course through the transverse mesocolon.
(c) True – the greater omentum descends from the greater curve of the stomach
     and proximal duodenum, passes inferiorly and then turns superiorly to insert
     into the transverse colon.

(d) The lesser omentum forms the anterior surface of the lesser sac.

(e) The inferior extent of the lesser omentum attaches to the porta hepatis.

10. Regarding the peritoneal ligaments:

(a) Between the two layers of the right coronary ligament is the bare area of the liver.

(b) The gastro-splenic ligament is a continuation of the lesser omentum from the stomach to the spleen.

(c) The falciform ligament contains the ligamentum venosum in its free edge.

(d) The phrenicocolic ligament is continuous with the splenorenal ligament.

(e) The hepatoduodenal ligament transports the portal triad.

11. In the anterior abdomen:

(a) The superficial fascia has a superficial layer that is continuous with the superficial perineal fascia.

(b) The paired rectus abdomini are separated by the linea alba.

(c) The rectus sheath is formed by the rectus muscles.

(d) The inguinal ligament is formed by the aponeurosis of the internal oblique muscle.

(e) The superior epigastric artery runs in the posterior rectus sheath.

12. In the abdomen:

(a) The foregut extends from the lower oesophagus to the second part of the duodenum.

(b) The outline of both psoas muscles is seen in the majority of plain radiographs.

(d) True – its free edge extends to the porta hepatis as the hepatoduodenal ligament.
(e) False – the superior extent of the lesser omentum is attached to the fissures for the porta hepatis and ligamentum venosum.

10.

(a) True – the liver in the bare area is attached to the diaphragm by areolar tissue and this area is continuous with the anterior pararenal space.
(b) False – this is a continuation of the greater omentum from the greater curve of the stomach to the spleen. It contains the short gastric and left gastroepiploic vessels.
(c) False – this carries the obliterated left umbilical vein (ligamentum teres) in its free edge. It is continuous with the fissure for the ligamentum venosum.
(d) True – and the transverse mesocolon (see question 6 (e)).
(e) True – this represents the thickened right edge of the lesser omentum. Behind it is the epiploic foramen leading into the lesser sac.

11.

(a) False – the deep layer of the superficial fascia passes inferomedially to form the superficial perineal fascia.
(b) True
(c) False – the aponeurosis of the oblique and transverse muscles of the anterior abdominal wall form the rectus sheath within which the rectus abdominis muscle is enclosed.
(d) False – the aponeurosis of the external oblique muscle forms a strong thick band – the inguinal ligament between the anterior superior iliac spine and the pubic tubercle.
(e) True – this is a branch of the internal thoracic (mammary artery), runs behind the rectus muscle and then pierces and supplies it. Inferiorly it anastomoses with the inferior epigastric artery, a branch of the external iliac artery.

12.

(a) False – the foregut extends from the pharynx to the second part of the duodenum.
(b) False – only seen in 48% of normal radiographs.

(c) In a plain radiograph the properitoneal fat lines seen in each flank represent the borders of the peritoneum.
(d) The cardiac orifice of the stomach is at the level of T10 vertebra.
(e) The right and left vagus nerves, oesophageal branches of the left gastric vessels are transmitted through the oesophageal hiatus in the diaphragm.

13. The oesophagus:

(a) has both striated and smooth muscle fibres in its lower third.
(b) is related to the left recurrent laryngeal nerve.
(c) is anterior to the right subclavian artery in the thorax.
(d) is related to the azygos vein and the pleura below T4.
(e) is posterior to the left main bronchus.

14. Regarding the oesophagus:

(a) The upper third is supplied by the inferior thyroid artery.
(b) The middle third is supplied by the branches of the aorta.
(c) The left gastric artery supplies the lower third.
(d) The lower third drains into the portal system.
(e) The upper oesophagus has lymphatic drainage to the mediastinal lymph nodes.

15. Regarding the gullet:

(a) Deglutition is best assessed by barium swallow examination using spot films.
(b) A high kV chest radiograph may show the right wall of the oesophagus better than low kV chest radiograph.

(c) True
(d) True
(e) True

13.

(a) False – the muscular layers of the oesophagus are the superficial longitudinal and inner circular layers. In the upper third the fibres are striated, in the middle third the muscles are both striated and smooth fibres and in the lower third there are only smooth muscle fibres.
(b) True – in the neck the left recurrent laryngeal nerve runs in the tracheo-oesophageal groove and the trachea is anterior to the oesophagus.
(c) False – though the oesophagus enters the thorax in the midline it deviates to the left of the midline. In the upper thorax, the left subclavian artery, aortic arch and upper part of descending aorta lie on its left.
(d) True – above T4 the oesophagus lies next to the pleura – forming the pleuro-oesophageal line.
(e) True – in the thorax from above downwards the trachea, left main bronchus, right pulmonary artery, left atrium and pericardium.

14.

(a) True – a branch of the subclavian artery.
(b) True
(c) True
(d) True – the left gastric vein drains the lower third into the portal system. The middle third drains into the azygos, therefore there is an important anastomosis between the azygos and portal system via the left gastric vein. The upper third drains into the brachiocephalic veins.
(e) False – the upper oesophagus has lymphatic drainage into the deep cervical nodes, the middle to the posterior mediastinal nodes of the coeliac group.

15.

(a) False – videofluoroscopy is used to assess the act of deglutition and provides anatomical information.
(b) True – this may demonstrate the right wall of the oesophagus and azygos vein as they are outlined by the lung – the azygo-oesophageal line.

(c) An oesophageal stricture is best assessed with the patient upright.
(d) The normal indentations of the oesophagus are seen anteriorly and to the left.
(e) The aberrant right subclavian artery with a left-sided arch of the aorta causes a posterior indentation of the oesophagus.

16. The stomach:

(a) is completely covered by peritoneum.
(b) is anterior to the left kidney.
(c) has a blood supply from all three branches of the coeliac axis.
(d) has a lymph drainage that follows the arterial supply.
(e) has areae gastricae which are longitudinal elevations of the mucosa.

17. Concerning the stomach:

(a) Ultrasound of the stomach is useful in the diagnosis of infantile pyloric stenosis.
(b) ^{111}In DTPA can be used to assess gastric emptying.
(c) The local spread of stomach tumours is best assessed by MRI.
(d) The anterior surface of the stomach can be differentiated from the posterior surface during a barium meal.
(e) The oesophagogastric junction is the 'B' ring or Schatzki ring.

(c) False – in the prone position the oesophagus is distended well and strictures which may be missed in the upright position are best seen.

(d) True – from above downwards these are as follows; where the pharynx joins the oesophagus, aortic arch, left main bronchus and where the oesophagus passes through the diaphragm.

(e) True – in a left-sided aortic arch the aberrant right subclavian artery is the last brachiocephalic branch and courses obliquely from the left to the right behind the oesophagus. The aberrant left main pulmonary artery produces an anterior indentation.

16.

(a) True – the lesser and greater omentum.

(b) True – and the left suprarenal gland, gastric surfaces of spleen and anterosuperior surface of the pancreas, the mesocolon and the transverse colon.

(c) True – the left gastric (from coeliac trunk) , right gastric (a branch of the common hepatic artery which arises from the coeliac artery), short gastric and left gastroepiploic arteries from the splenic artery (a branch of the coeliac trunk), right gastroepiploic artery from the gastroduodenal artery (a branch of the hepatic artery).

(d) True – and drains into the coeliac lymph nodes.

(e) False – these are small nodular elevations of the mucosal surface which measure 2–3 mm seen particularly in the gastric antrum.

17.

(a) True – as well as appendicitis, and intussusception in children.

(b) True

(c) True – endoluminal ultrasound is probably best to assess the stomach wall.

(d) True – in the supine position, barium pools around the posterior rugal folds due to gravity.

(e) False – the lower end of the oesophagus is dilated to form the vestibule, just above the oesophagogastric junction (mucosal junction between the oeosphagus and stomach – the 'Z' line). The upper limit of the vestibule is the 'A' ring and the lower limit as the 'B' ring or Schatzki ring which is usually below the diaphragm.

18. Regarding the duodenum:

(a) This C-shaped tube is wholly retroperitoneal.
(b) The first part runs upwards, forwards and to the right.
(c) The duodenal cap has the same rugal pattern as the pylorus.
(d) The IVC lies directly behind the first part of the duodenum.
(e) The head of the pancreas is inferior to the first part of the duodenum.

19. Regarding the duodenum:

(a) The second part is anterior to the hilum of the right kidney.
(b) The ampulla of Vater is in the posteromedial aspect of the second part.
(c) The fundus of the gall bladder lies anterior to the second part.
(d) The superior mesenteric vessels are posterior to the third part.
(e) The left psoas muscle is posterior to the terminal portion of the third part.

20. Regarding the duodenum:

(a) The duodenojejunal junction is at the level of the second lumbar vertebra.
(b) The duodenal junction is held by the ligament of Treitz, a peritoneal fold that ascends to the left crus of the diaphragm.
(c) The mucosa of the first part of the duodenum is broken up into circular folds – 'plica circularis'.
(d) The duodenal lymphatic drainage is primarily to the coeliac nodes.
(e) The duodenum is predominantly supplied by the coeliac axis.

18.

(a) False – the first inch (2.5 cm) of the duodenum is intraperitoneal. The remainder is retroperitoneal as it is covered only anteriorly by peritoneum.
(b) False – it runs upwards, backwards and to the right from the pylorus. Hence, the right anterior oblique position is needed to open out the loop formed by the first part with the second part of the duodenum. (The patient 's right side is half-way off the table with an overcouch tube.)
(c) True – this is the first 2 cm of the duodenum which is slightly conical in shape and is between the folds of the greater and lesser omentum.
(d) False – the portal vein lies between the first part of the duodenum and the IVC posteriorly.
(e) True

19.

(a) True
(b) True
(c) True – and right lobe of liver.
(d) False – exit the neck of the pancreas and run over the third part.
(e) False – the right ureter, right psoas, IVC and aorta are the posterior relations of the third part of the duodenum from the right to left. The fourth part lies on the left psoas muscle.

20.

(a) True
(b) False – it ascends to the right crus of the diaphragm. An abnormal position of this ligament indicates mal-rotation.
(c) False – the mucosa of the first part of the duodenum is smooth. The rest of the small bowel is broken into the 'plica circularis'.
(d) False – the proximal duodenum is drained via pancreatico-duodenal nodes to the gastroduodenal nodes and to the coeliac nodes. The distal duodenum drains to the pancreatico-duodenal nodes which drain into the superior mesenteric nodes.
(e) False – dual supply from SMA and coeliac axis – hence the difficulty in controlling bleeding from an eroding duodenal ulcer.

21. In the small intestine:

(a) The transition from jejunum to the ileum takes place gradually.
(b) A Meckel's diverticulum occurs in 2% of the population.
(c) The small bowel mesentery is anterior to the right gonadal vessels.
(d) The plica circulares are most prominent in the terminal ileum.
(e) ^{99m} Technetium-labelled colloid is used to detect Meckel's diverticulum.

22. Regarding the large intestine:

(a) The lateral cutaneous nerve of the thigh is posterior to the caecum.
(b) An appendicolith is seen in 15% of the normal population.
(c) The ascending and descending colon are covered anteriorly and laterally by peritoneum.
(d) The third part of the duodenum lies posteriorly to the transverse colon.
(e) The proximal third of the transverse colon is supplied by the middle colic artery and the remaining two-thirds by the left colic artery.

23. Regarding the large intestine:

(a) The sigmoid colon is retroperitoneal.
(b) The marginal artery of Drummond is a single arterial trunk formed by anastomoses of arteries around the inner border of the colon.
(c) Taenia coli are thickenings of the longitudinal muscle layers.
(d) The colon has sacculations due to the mucosal folds.
(e) The appendices epiploicae are sparse in the sigmoid colon.

21.

(a) True

(b) True – it is found in the ileum, on the antimesenteric border. Its blind end may contain gastric mucosa, liver or pancreatic tissue.

(c) True – from left to right posteriorly are the fourth part of duodenum, aorta, IVC, right gonadal vessels, the right ureter and psoas muscle.

(d) False – they become less prominent and less numerous in the ileum until at the terminal ileum, they are almost entirely absent.

(e) False – Meckel's diverticulum containing gastric mucosa is detected using ^{99m}Technetium pertechnetate. Occult bleeding in the small bowel is detected using ^{99m}Tc labelled with colloid or red cells. Active bleeding at a rate of more than 0.5 ml per minute is required to enable detection at angiography.

22.

(a) True – and the femoral nerve, the psoas and iliacus muscles.

(b) True – in patients with acute abdominal pain their presence indicates a 90% chance of appendicitis.

(c) True – this binds it to the posterior abdominal wall.

(d) False – it is the second part of the duodenum.

(e) False – the proximal two-thirds is supplied by the middle colic artery (branch of the superior mesenteric artery). The distal one-third is supplied by the ascending branch of the left colic artery (from the inferior mesenteric artery).

23.

(a) False – the sigmoid colon is completely invested in peritoneum. It is attached to the posterior pelvic wall by the fan-shaped sigmoid meso-colon.

(b) True

(c) True – these are three narrow bands present on the outer wall of the colon, they converge on the appendix proximally and the rectum distally.

(d) False – the taeniae are shorter than the colon. Therefore the colon is thrown into sacculations which give the appearance of haustra on radiographs.

(e) False – they are sparse in the caecum and rectum and most numerous in the sigmoid colon. Herniation of mucous membrane through the appendices apiplocae leads to formation of diverticula.

24. Regarding the large intestine:

(a) The gas-filled large bowel on plain radiographs demonstrates the haustral pattern of incomplete septations.
(b) In Chilaiditi syndrome there is hepatodiaphragmatic interposition of the colon.
(c) The upper third of the rectum is covered in front and on both sides by peritoneum.
(d) The rectum is supplied by branches of the internal iliac artery.
(e) There is a portosystemic anastomosis between the middle and inferior rectal veins.

25. Regarding the rectum and anal canal:

(a) The lower two-thirds of the rectum drains into the internal iliac nodes.
(b) The anal canal is about 3 cm long.
(c) The upper part of the vagina is anterior to the anal canal.
(d) The lymphatic drainage of the anal canal is to the internal iliac nodes.
(e) The superior rectal artery supplies the upper half of the anal canal.

26. Regarding the rectum and anal canal:

(a) The anal canal is well visualized during a barium enema.
(b) During defaecating proctography the dynamics of rectal evacuation and position of the anorectal junction is evaluated.
(c) MRI is the investigation of choice to detect anal fistulae.
(d) The musculus submucosa ani has a high signal intensity compared to fat and submucosa on T_1-weighted MRI.
(e) The subcutaneous fibres of the external sphincter have a high signal on T_1-weighted MRI.

24.

(a) True – the valvulae conniventis of the small bowel are complete.

(b) True – this is an asymptomatic condition, which can mimic the appearance of free intraperitoneal air and lead to unnecessary laparotomy.

(c) True – the middle third is covered in front only and the lower third is uncovered.

(d) True – the superior rectal (branch of inferior mesenteric), middle rectal (branch of internal iliac), inferior rectal (branch of internal pudendal) and median sacral artery (continuation of the aorta) supply the rectum.

(e) False – the superior rectal (a tributary of the inferior mesenteric which drains into the portal vein) forms an important portosystemic anastomosis with the middle rectal vein and inferior rectal vein (branches of internal iliac and internal pudendal veins).

25.

(a) True – the lymphatic drainage follows vascular supply. The upper two-thirds drains into the inferior mesenteric nodes.

(b) True – and perpendicular to the rectum. This is important to remember when inserting a rectal tube. The tip of the tube has to be angled perpendicular and upwards after the first few centimetres into the anal canal to avoid hitting the anterior rectal wall, which is painful.

(c) False – the lower part.

(d) False – the lymph from the upper half of the anal canal drains into the inferior mesenteric nodes. The lower half drains into the superficial inguinal nodes.

(e) True – the inferior rectal artery supplies the lower half.

26.

(a) False – the enema tube position prevents this.

(b) True – the anorectal junction at rest is just above the level of the ischial tuberosities. During evacuation the pelvic floor descends and the anorectal angle widens from 90° to 115°.

(c) True

(d) False – the musculus submucosa ani is a fascial extension of the longitudinal muscle coat of the rectum which inserts into the mucocutaneous junction (the Hilton's white line). This has a low signal intensity compared to the high signal fat and submucosa on T_1-W MRI.

(e) False

27. In vascular imaging of the gastrointestinal tract:

(a) Digital subtraction angiography may be degraded by patient movement.
(b) The coeliac axis arises from the aorta at the level of T12 and L1 interspace.
(c) The coeliac axis may be compressed by the median arcuate ligament preventing antegrade flow of blood.
(d) The left gastric artery runs upwards to the cardia.
(e) The coeliac axis is inferior to the lesser omentum.

28. Regarding the branches of the coeliac axis:

(a) The splenic artery is intraperitoneal during most of its course.
(b) The transverse pancreatic artery is a branch of the left gastric artery.
(c) The arteria pancreatica magna is a branch of the dorsal pancreatic artery.
(d) The left gastro-epiploic artery arises from the terminal portion of the main splenic artery.
(e) The left epiploic artery is a branch of the left gastro-epiploic artery.

29. Concerning the hepatic arteries:

(a) The common hepatic artery usually lies to the left of the common bile duct and anterior to the portal vein.
(b) The right hepatic artery usually crosses the common hepatic duct anteriorly.

27.

(a) True – in abdominal imaging bowel movement and respiration can worsen this. However this can be overcome by using anti-peristaltic agents and by obtaining multiple 'mask' images during the angiographic run whilst the patient is breathing, before contrast is injected.
(b) True
(c) True – resulting in enlargement of collateral vessels arising from the superior or inferior mesenteric arteries.
(d) True – in 3% it arises directly from the aorta. It gives off cardio-oesphageal, anastomosing branches to the terminal branches of the right gastric and short gastric arteries. In 25% of individuals the left lobe of the liver is supplied by an aberrant left hepatic artery arising from the left gastric artery.
(e) False – it lies above the pancreas and splenic veins, below the left lobe of the liver, on its left is the cardia of the stomach and in front is the lesser omentum.

28.

(a) False – retroperitoneal most of its course and enters the lienorenal ligament before entering the spleen.
(b) False – the transverse pancreatic artery is a branch of the dorsal pancreatic artery, which arises from the proximal splenic artery.
(c) False – this is a branch of the mid-portion of the splenic artery and is usually the largest branch to the body of the pancreas.
(d) True – or from one of its terminal branches. It descends along the greater curvature of the stomach to form the 'arcus arteriosus ventriculi inferior of Hyrtl' with the right gastro-epiploic artery.
(e) True – the left epiploic artery, a branch of the left gastro-epiploic is located in the posterior layers of the greater omentum below the transverse colon. It anastomoses with the right epiploic to form the arcus epiploicus magnus of Barkow.

29.

(a) True – its first major branch is the gastroduodenal artery after which it continues as the proper hepatic artery and divides into the right and left hepatic arteries.
(b) False – usually posteriorly.

(c) The middle hepatic artery supplies the caudate lobe.
(d) The left hepatic artery supplies the left lobe segments.
(e) In approximately 25% of individuals the entire hepatic arterial supply arises from the superior mesenteric artery (SMA).

30. Regarding the arteries of the upper abdomen:

(a) The cystic artery to the gall bladder usually arises from the right hepatic artery.
(b) The right gastric artery is a branch of the superior mesenteric artery.
(c) The gastroduodenal artery (GDA) arises usually from the right hepatic artery.
(d) The proximal GDA descends anterior to the first part of the duodenum.
(e) The GDA terminates into the right gastro-epiploic and anterior superior pancreaticoduodenal arteries.

31. Regarding the blood supply to the pancreas:

(a) The retroduodenal artery forms an arcade to supply the posterior surface of the entire duodenum and part of the pancreatic head.
(b) The inferior pancreatico-duodenal artery may arise from a proximal jejunal artery.
(c) The transverse pancreatic artery may arise from the anterior superior pancreatico-duodenal artery.
(d) The blood flow in the arterial tree is usually unidirectional.
(e) The majority of the blood supply to the pancreas is derived from the dorsal pancreatic artery.

32. The superior mesenteric artery (SMA):

(a) arises from the anterior surface of the aorta at about the level of L1.
(b) gives rise to the dorsal pancreatic artery.
(c) gives rise to the middle colic artery inferior to the uncinate process.
(d) gives rise to the right colic artery in a third of individuals.
(e) gives rise to the inferior pancreatico-duodenal artery in the majority of cases.

(c)   False – It supplies the quadrate lobe – segment IV.

(d)   True – runs in the fossa for the ligamentum venosum.

(e)   False – in 20% of individuals all or part of the hepatic arterial supply arises from the SMA, of these 10–12% will be replaced by right hepatic artery from the SMA, 4–6% from an accessory right hepatic artery from the coeliac axis. In 2.5% the entire hepatic arterial supply arises from the SMA.

30.

(a)   True

(b)   False – arises from the proper or left hepatic arteries in about equal proportions. It supplies the pylorus and courses along the lesser curve to anastomose with the left gastic artery.

(c)   False – In 75% of cases from the common hepatic artery.

(d)   False – behind the first part of the duodenum. Erosion of the duodenum by an ulcer can produce torrential bleeding and death if the GDA is involved. In this position the GDA is anterior to the pancreas.

(e)   True

31.

(a)   True – the head has a dual blood supply. The superior pancreatico-duodenal from the GDA and inferior pancreatico-duodenal from the SMA, both of which have anterior and posterior divisions forming extensive anastomoses.

(b)   True – most commonly from the SMA.

(c)   True – in 10%. The transverse pancreatic artery is usually (75%) a branch of the dorsal pancreatic artery.

(d)   False – numerous anastomoses allow multi-directional flow.

(e)   False – the majority of the blood supply is from the splenic artery.

32.

(a)   True – lies posterior to the body of the pancreas and splenic vein.

(b)   True – or it arises from the SMA's first jejunal branch.

(c)   True – which enters the transverse mesocolon.

(d)   True – Right colic is absent in 2% and arises most frequently from the middle colic artery.

(e)   False – in 40% it arises as a single trunk from the SMA. In at least half of all individuals the common trunk or one of the anterior or posterior divisions arise from the first or second jejunal artery. This is important to bear in mind during selective catheterization of IPDA.

33. Regarding the arteries of the lower abdomen:

(a) The inferior mesenteric artery arises from the anterior or left antero-lateral aspect of the aorta at the level of L1.
(b) The left colic artery anastomosis with the middle colic artery.
(c) The superior rectal artery is the terminal artery of the inferior mesenteric artery.
(d) The middle and inferior rectal arteries anastomose with the superior rectal artery.
(e) The marginal artery of Dwight runs close to the distal large bowel from which the vasa recta arise.

34. Regarding the portal venous system:

(a) Direct portography may be achieved by a transjugular transhepatic approach.
(b) The splenic and superior mesenteric vein join to form the main portal vein.
(c) The extra hepatic portal vein lies anterior to the common bile duct.
(d) The right portal vein supplies the caudate lobe.
(e) The umbilical (distal) portion of the left portal vein supplies the lateral segments 2 and 3 and the inferior portion of segment 4.

35. Regarding the venous drainage of the gut:

(a) The superior mesenteric vein usually lies to the left of the superior mesenteric artery.
(b) The posterior superior pancreatico-duodenal vein drains into the main portal vein.
(c) The inferior mesenteric vein drains into the splenic vein in majority of individuals.
(d) The left gastric vein drains into the confluence of the splenic and superior mesenteric vein.
(e) The venous arcade formed by the epiploic veins serve as a collateral venous return from the spleen.

36. Regarding hepatobiliary imaging:

(a) CT arterio-portography (CTAP) is undertaken by catheterizing the SMA prior to CT scanning.

33.

(a) False – L 3.
(b) True
(c) True
(d) True – they are derived from the internal iliac artery.
(e) False – the marginal artery of Dwight is situated close to the small bowel and the marginal artery of Drummond is close to the large bowel. The artery of Drummond may hypertrophy significantly when one of the main visceral arteries is compromised.

34.

(a) True – or puncture of the spleen, percutaneous portal vein puncture or through the umbilcal vein.
(b) True – behind the neck of the pancreas.
(c) False – the common bile duct(CBD) and hepatic artery are anterior to the portal vein. The CBD is to the right and hepatic artery lies to the left.
(d) False – the caudate lobe is supplied by the left portal vein.
(e) True – the obliterated umbilical vein is patent in the presence of portal hypertension, courses vertically from the umbilical portion of the left portal vein in the falciform ligament to the anterior abdominal wall.

35.

(a) False – SMV lies to the right of the SMA.
(b) True
(c) False – drains into the splenic vein in 40%, into the confluence of the SMV and splenic vein in 30% and into the SMV in 30%.
(d) True – into the splenic vein in 15%, into the main portal vein in 25%.
(e) True – the epiploic veins are tributaries of the gastro-epiploic veins.

36.

(a) True – contrast is injected at 2 ml/second into the SMA which passes into the capillary bed of the mid gut and then into the portal vein. CT scanning during the portal venous phase outlines the portal vein, portal venous perfusion and hepatic veins.

(b) CTAP enables better delineation of metastases than conventional CT.
(c) In magnetic resonance cholangiopancreatography (MRCP) bile has a low signal.
(d) Magnetic resonance cholangiopancreatography uses heavily T_2-weighted sequences.
(e) The liver parenchyma exhibits high signal on MRCP sequences.

37. Concerning the adult liver:

(a) It is anterior to the upper pole of the right kidney and suprarenal gland.
(b) On ultrasound it has a slightly increased echogenicity compared with kidney.
(c) The walls of the hepatic veins are bright compared with those of the portal vein and its branches.
(d) The intrahepatic bile ducts are usually clearly seen parallel to the portal vein.
(e) On non-enhanced CT the liver has a higher attenuation than the spleen.

38. Regarding the liver:

(a) Primary and secondary liver tumours derive their blood supply from the hepatic artery.
(b) The segmental anatomy of the liver relates to the hepatic arterial, portal and biliary drainage to the liver.
(c) On axial imaging the caudate lobe (segment 1) is posterior and to the right of the IVC.
(d) Segments II, IVa, VIII, VII are above the portal vein in an anticlockwise fashion on axial CT.
(e) Segments III, IVb, V, VI are below the portal vein in a clockwise fashion on axial CT.

39. In the upper abdomen:

(a) The caudate lobe of the liver lies in the greater sac.
(b) The gall bladder is posterior to the porta hepatis.

(b) True – most hepatic tumours are supplied by the hepatic artery. CTAP produces dense enhancement of normal liver parenchyma and no enhancement of lesions supplied by hepatic artery.

(c) False – high signal.

(d) True

(e) False

37.

(a) True – the upper pole of right kidney, suprarenal gland and distal IVC are related directly to the liver and have no peritoneal coverings. Therefore free fluid cannot be seen anterior to the upper pole of the right kidney except in patients who have undergone liver transplantation.

(b) True

(c) False – the opposite is True

(d) False – the 'shotgun' sign when the bile ducts are of similar calibre and parallel to the portal vein indicates that there is intrahepatic biliary duct dilatation. However this sign may be seen in portal hypertension when there is compensatory enlargement of the branches of the hepatic artery, alongside those of the portal vein. Colour doppler will distinguish ducts from vessels.

(e) True – standard settings for upper abdomen are a window level of 40 to 60 HU and window width of 350 to 400 HU using 10 mm contiguous cuts. The relative density of the liver is 60 HU.

38.

(a) True

(b) True

(c) True

(d) True

(e) False

39.

(a) False – the omental reflections divide the caudate from the quadrate lobe. The caudate lobe lies in the lesser sac and the quadrate lobe lies within the greater sac.

(b) False – the gall bladder fossa is anterior to the porta hepatis.

(c) The hepatic artery is anterior to the portal vein.
(d) The hepatic vein tributaries run with those of the hepatic artery and bile ducts in the portal triad.
(e) Behind the first part of the duodenum the common bile duct is anterior to the IVC.

40. Regarding the gall bladder:

(a) The gall bladder indents the posterior aspect of the first part of the duodenum.
(b) The cystic duct passes anterior to the right hepatic artery.
(c) On ultrasound, the neck of the gall bladder and the cystic duct are echogenic.
(d) The Phrygian cap is the fundus folded back upon the body of the gall bladder.
(e) Lymph drainage mainly follows the common bile duct to the liver.

41. Concerning the pancreas:

(a) The gland is angled inferiorly from right to left.
(b) Most of the gland is posterior to the lesser sac.
(c) The uncinate process is superior to the origin of the superior mesenteric artery.
(d) The gastroduodenal artery is anterior to the head of the pancreas.
(e) On ultrasound the pancreas may be hyperechoic compared with the liver.

42. The spleen:

(a) lies posterior to the axillary line adjacent to the ninth and eleventh ribs.
(b) on ultrasound should measure no more than 14 cm in its longest axis.
(c) is formed from the splenic diverticulum.
(d) takes up ^{99m}Tc denatured red blood cells.
(e) enhances homogeneously in the early arterial phase of contrast-enhanced CT.

(c) True
(d) False – the radicles of the portal vein, hepatic artery and bile duct run in the portal triads.
(e) True – this is the middle third of the CBD, The lower third of the CBD runs inferiorly and to the right, behind the head of pancreas. This portion of the CBD grooves or tunnels the head of the pancreas and is anterior to the right renal vein.

40.

(a) False – anterior aspect of first part of duodenum.
(b) True
(c) True – hence mistaken for gallstones.
(d) True
(e) True – some lymph from the gall bladder flows directly into the liver. This is important in malignancy of the gall bladder as it may be necessary to resect local segments of the liver with the gall bladder tumour.

41.

(a) False – it is angled superiorly from right to left.
(b) True
(c) False – anterior to the origin of SMA . The left renal vein is posterior.
(d) False – GDA is anterior to the neck of the pancreas.
(e) True – with increasing age the pancreas becomes more echogenic due to progressive accumulation of fat (see question 7 under 'Breast').

42.

(a) True
(b) True
(c) False – it is of mesenchymal origin and is formed by numerous splenunculi which fuse. Ten per cent of unfused or accessory splenunculi are demonstrated on USG or CT, usually in the region of the hilum or lienorenal ligament.
(d) True – post splenectomy to detect residual splenic tissue.
(e) False – the intrasplenic blood supply is inconsistent. This is appreciated on CT as inhomogeneous enhancement in the early arterial phase.

43. The following are recognized anastomotic sites between portal and systemic circulations:

(a) Azygos and left gastric veins.
(b) Superior rectal and middle rectal veins.
(c) Portal and hepatic veins.
(d) Ovarian and mesenteric veins.
(e) Left renal and splenic vein.

43.

(a) True
(b) True
(c) True
(d) False
(e) False

Module 4

Genito-urinary and adrenal (renal tract and retroperitoneum)*

A. Doss and M. J. Bull

1. Regarding the development of the urinary tract:

(a) The metanepheric duct develops from a diverticulum at the end of the mesonephric duct.
(b) The metanephros differentiates from the ureteric bud to develop into the kidney.
(c) The metanephric duct develops into the ureter,
(d) The metanephros develps into the glomeruli and the proximal part of the renal duct system.
(e) The collecting system of the kidney is derived from endoderm.

2. Regarding the kidney:

(a) It ascends from the pelvis during development.
(b) An aberrant renal artery may run to the kidney from the common iliac artery.
(c) Fusion of the metanephric masses across the midline results in a duplex kidney.
(d) Congenital absence of one kidney occurs in about one in 100 births.
(e) The primitive urogenital sinus gives rise to the bladder, urethra and vestibule of the vagina.

3. In the renal tract:

(a) A high kV radiograph optimizes the detection of calcification.
(b) Perirenal fat allows the renal outline to be seen on plain films.
(c) The ureters are projected over the tips of the transverse processes of L2 to L5.
(d) On tomograms the renal upper pole is posterior to the lower pole.
(e) Prone views aid mid ureteric filling during an IVU.

---

* From *Applied Radiological Anatomy*. 'The renal tract and retroperitoneum'.

Genito-urinary and adrenal (renal tract and retroperitoneum)*

ANSWERS

1.

(a) True – also known as the ureteric bud.
(b) True
(c) True – and the renal pelvis, calyces and collecting tubules.
(d) True
(e) False – from mesoderm.

2.

(a) True – as the ureteric outgrowth lengthens, the kidney is situated more and more cranially.
(b) True – as the kidney ascends from the pelvis, it gets its blood sequentially from the middle sacral, common iliac arteries and finally from the aorta. Hence one of these arteries may persist in later life.
(c) False – this is a horseshoe kidney. On ultrasound, difficulty in defining the lower poles of the kidneys, should alert the sonographer to this variant.
(d) False – 1 in 2400 births.
(e) True

3.

(a) False – a low KV radiograph.
(b) True
(c) True – and over the sacroiliac joints, and within the pelvis over a course which runs laterally to the ischial spines and medially towards the bladder.
(d) True – due to orientation of the kidneys to the lumbar lordosis. The whole length of the kidney is seen with slight caudal angulation of the X-ray tube.
(e) True

---

* From *Applied Radiological Anatomy*: 'The renal tract and retroperitoneum'.

4. Regarding the kidneys:

(a) On ultrasound of the kidney the cortex is echopoor compared with the medulla.
(b) On T_1-W MRI the cortex is of higher signal than the medulla.
(c) They usually lie between T12 and L3 vertebra.
(d) Corticomedullary differentiation is appreciated on a DMSA scan.
(e) The upper poles lie more laterally than the lower poles.

5. In the kidney:

(a) The right kidney is usually larger by about 1.5 cm than the left.
(b) The columns of Bertin extend medially within the substance of the kidney separating the medulla into pyramids.
(c) Compound calyces are less efficient at preventing intrarenal reflux of urine.
(d) The renal arteries arise from the aorta at the superior margin of T12.
(e) The right renal artery is posterior to the IVC.

6. In the kidney:

(a) The anterior division of the renal artery supplies both upper and lower portions of the kidney.
(b) The segmental branches divide into interlobar arteries between the pyramids.
(c) The arcuate arteries anastomose extensively with each other at the base of the pyramids.
(d) The renal vein is anterior to the renal pelvis.
(e) The left renal vein is anterior to the aorta.

7. Regarding the fascial planes and spaces around the kidney:

(a) The perirenal fat is surrounded by Gerota's fascia.
(b) The anterior pararenal space lies between the anterior leaf of Gerota's fascia and the posterior peritoneum.

4.

(a) True – cortex is echopoor and medulla is echobright. This is cortico-medullary differentiation and fat within the renal sinus is very bright.
(b) True
(c) True
(d) False – Dimercaptosuccinic acid (DMSA) scintigrams give information on renal scarring and renal function. DTPA (diethylene triamine pentacetic acid) or mercaptocetyl triglycine (MAG3) scans quantify renal function and provide structural information, e.g. reflux of urine from the bladder into the ureter.
(e) False – upper poles lie more medially and posteriorly than lower poles (see question 3(d)).

5.

(a) False
(b) True
(c) True – and therefore are incriminated in the aetiology of reflux nephropathy (chronic pyelonephritis).
(d) False – superior margin of L2, immediately caudal to the origin of the SMA.
(e) True

6.

(a) True – the posterior division supplies the upper and mid-portion of the posterior aspect of the kidney.
(b) True
(c) False – they form individual arcs which do not anastomose.
(d) True
(e) True – and receives the inferior phrenic vein, the gonadal and suprarenal vein on the left. There are no extra-renal tributaries to the right renal vein.

7.

(a) True – Gerota's fascia has an anterior and posterior leaf.
(b) True – this space extends across the midline and encases the pancreas, duodenum and both ascending and descending colon.

(c) The posterior pararenal space lies between the kidneys and Gerota's fascia.
(d) The two leaves of Gerota's fascia fuse to form the lateral conal fascia.
(e) The suprarenal gland is outside the peri-renal space.

8. The ureter:

(a) shows narrowing at the pelvi-ureteric junction, when it crosses the iliac vessels at the pelvic brim and at the vesico-ureteric junction.
(b) on the right is crossed by the second part of the duodenum, gonadal, right colic and ileocolic vessels.
(c) in the male passes posterior to the seminal vesicle.
(d) in the female passes just superior to the uterine artery.
(e) from the upper moiety in complete duplication opens in an ectopic location.

9. Regarding the urinary tract:

(a) Renal duplication is commoner in females than males.
(b) A ureterocele when associated with duplication usually affects the ectopic ureter.
(c) In fetal lobulation the divisions overlie a calyx.
(d) A pancake kidney results from fusion of two ectopic pelvic kidneys.
(e) A horseshoe kidney usually lies higher than the normal kidney.

(c) False – between the posterior leaf of Gerota's fascia and the muscles of the posterior abdominal wall. Laterally the space is continuous with the extraperitoneal fat. Therefore, using an anterior abdominal wall incision an operation on retroperitoneal structures can be performed.

(d) True – this passes lateral to the colon and medial to the posterior renal space.

(e) False – exact location is in debate (see question 10).

8.

(a) True

(b) True – and root of the mesentery and terminal ileum. As the aorta is left sided the ureter is less oblique over the right common iliac artery compared to the left. Thus a greater length of the right ureter is compressed during pregnancy leading to pyelonephritis on this side.

(c) False – anterosuperior to the seminal vesicle. The ureter is usually lateral to the IVC – except in a retrocaval ureter.

(d) False – inferior and here it is in danger during a hysterectomy.

(e) True – the ureter from the lower moiety inserts obliquely and predisposes to reflux and that of the upper moiety leads to ureterocele and obstruction.

9.

(a) True – prevalence of about 2%.

(b) True – a ureterocele is a dilatation of the intramural part of the ureter due to narrowing of the ureteric orifice.

(c) False – in cortical scarring, the loss of cortex overlies a calyx. In fetal lobulation the divisions lie between calyces.

(d) True – pelvic kidneys derive their blood supply from the internal iliac artery.

(e) False – lies lower. The ascent of the horseshoe kidney is prevented by the inferior mesenteric artery. It occurs in 1 in 100 individuals. The lower pole of a normally situated kidney may fuse with the upper pole of an ectopic kidney – a crossed fused ectopia. Despite abnormal migration of the kidneys the suprarenals almost always lie in their usual sites apart from assuming a discoid shape, due to the absence of the renal impression in utero.

10. The suprarenal gland(s):

(a) at birth are the same size as the kidney.
(b) are separated from the kidney by a thin layer of peri-renal fat and lie at the superior margin of the peri-renal fascia.
(c) have limbs that are usually no more than the size of the adjacent diaphragmatic crus.
(d) on the right is anterior to the IVC.
(e) on the left is anterior to the lesser sac.

11. Regarding the suprarenal glands:

(a) The superior suprarenal artery is a branch of the inferior phrenic artery.
(b) The suprarenal artery proper is a branch of the corresponding renal arteries.
(c) The right suprarenal vein drains into the right renal vein.
(d) The arteries to the suprarenal gland arise at about the level of L1/L2 intervertebral disc.
(e) Islands of suprarenal cortical tissue may be found in the broad ligament.

12. The IVC:

(a) is formed at the level of L5 by the confluences of the right and left common iliac veins.
(b) At the level of the diaphragm, is separated from the aorta by the right crus of the diaphragm and oesophagus.
(c) pierces the central tendon of the diaphragm at the level of T12.
(d) drains the left renal vein adjacent to the uncinate process of the pancreas.
(e) drain the segmental lumbar veins.

13. Regarding the lymphatic system:

(a) The internal structure of nodes can sometimes be assessed on high resolution CT.

10.

(a) False – at birth they are about one-third the size of the kidney and atrophy until the second year of life after which slow growth occurs until pubery to reach adult size – about one-thirtieth the size of the kidney.
(b) True
(c) True
(d) False – posterior to the IVC and right lobe of the liver.
(e) False

11.

(a) True
(b) False – a branch of the aorta, it gives rise to the middle suprarenal artery. The renal arteries give rise to the inferior suprarenal arteries.
(c) False – the left suprarenal vein drains into the left renal vein. The right suprarenal vein drains directly into the IVC.
(d) True
(e) True – and epididymis and spermatic cord.

12.

(a) True
(b) True
(c) False – at T8.
(d) True
(e) True – spread of infection or tumour from the pelvis to the vertebral column is due to the ascending lumbar veins. The ascending lumbar veins connect the segmental lumbar veins which drain the vertebral venous plexuses into the IVC, and extend as far caudally as the lateral sacral veins and iliolumbar veins.

13.

(a) False – the internal structure of nodes can never be seen. Lymph nodes of 0.5–1 cm (normal size) can be detected, but the normal nodes cannot be discerned from the abnormal ones of this size.
(b) True
(c) True

(b) Nodes of more than 1cm in the external iliac territory are often normal.
(c) Nodes of 1cm on short axis in the retrocrural on left gastric territories are usually abnormal.
(d) Lymphography is the method of choice to visualize the internal iliac, hepatic and pre-aortic nodes.
(e) The cisterna chyli extends from the bifurcation of the aorta to just below the diaphragm.

14. Regarding the diaphragm:

(a) In the midline the crura join to form the lateral arcuate ligament.
(b) The fascia overlying the psoas muscle is thickened and gives origin to the diaphragm.
(c) The IVC passes through the most posterior of the diaphragmatic openings.
(d) The aorta enters the thorax anterior to the crura.
(e) The oeosphagus passes through the muscular part of the diaphragm in the region of the right crus.

(d) False – these group of nodes are not visualized on lymphography. High quality CT has almost completely replaced this technique.

(e) False – it is 6 cm long anterior to L1 and L2 posterior to the right crus of the diaphragm. It passes through the retrocrural space with the aorta to become the thoracic duct.

14.

(a) False – the median arcuate ligament which is a tendinous structure in the midline.

(b) True – this is the medial arcuate ligament. The lateral arcuate ligament is fascia overlying the quadratus lumborum muscles.

(c) False – the IVC pierces the central tendinous part of the diaphragm and is patent in all phases of respiration. It is the most anterior of the three openings.

(d) False – the aorta passes posterior to the median arcuate ligament in the retrocrural space. The rectrocrural space is bounded laterally by the crura, anteriorly by their fused median arcuate ligament and posteriorly by the vertebral body of T12.

(e) True – at the level of T10 with the right and left vagus nerves, oesophageal branches of the left gastric vessels and lymphatics draining the lower third of the oesophagus.

Pelvis*

A. Doss and M. J. Bull

1. Concerning the pelvic floor:

(a) The pelvic diaphragm is inferior to the superficial muscles of the perineum.
(b) The pelvic diaphragm is formed by levator ani and coccygeus muscles.
(c) The perineal aspect of the levator ani forms the medial wall of the ischiorectal fossa.
(d) The urogenital diaphragm is pierced by the urethra in both sexes.
(e) To the fibromuscular perineal body attach the anal sphincter and levator ani muscles.

2. Concerning the nerves of the pelvis:

(a) The sacral plexus is anterior to the piriformis muscle.
(b) The sciatic nerve can be visualized by CT and MRI as it passes through the greater sciatic foramen.
(c) The pudendal nerve leaves the pelvis through the lesser sciatic foramen to enter the perineum.
(d) The obturator nerve runs lateral to the psoas in the pelvis.
(e) The femoral nerve passes into the thigh under the inguinal ligament.

3. In the pelvis:

(a) The umbilical artery anastomoses with the inferior epigastric artery in the adult.
(b) The external iliac artery passes under the inguinal ligament to become the common femoral artery.
(c) The middle rectal artery is a branch of the internal pudendal artery.
(d) The obturator artery usually arises from the external iliac artery.
(e) A persistent sciatic artery may replace the superficial femoral artery.

---

* From *Applied Radiological Anatomy*. 'The pelvis'.

Pelvis*

ANSWERS

1.

(a) False – the pelvic diaphragm is superior to the superficial perineal muscles.
(b) True
(c) True
(d) True – and by the vagina in the female.
(e) True – and transverse perineal and bulbospongiosus muscles.

2.

(a) True
(b) True – the largest nerve in the body.
(c) False – the sacrospinous ligament and the sacrotuberous ligament form the superior and postero-inferior borders of the lesser sciatic foramen, respectively. The internal pudendal artery and pudendal nerve exit the pelvis through the greater sciatic foramen and enter the perineum through the lesser sciatic foramen.
(d) False – it runs medial to the psoas, and then along the lateral pelvic wall, lies posteromedial to the common iliac vein to enter the obturator canal.
(e) True

3.

(a) False – this is the first branch of the internal iliac artery in the fetus which persists as the medial umbilical ligament. This may be recognized in the presence of pneumoperitoneum.
(b) True
(c) False – the middle rectal artery is a branch of the anterior division of the internal iliac artery.
(d) False – it usually arises from the anterior division of the internal iliac artery in 75% of individuals. It may arise from the inferior epigastric artery in 25%.
(e) True – in less than 1% of individuals there is an enlarged inferior gluteal artery (branch of the anterior division) which represents persistent fetal vascular supply to the lower limbs.

* From *Applied Radiological Anatomy*: 'The pelvis'.

4. In the pelvis:

(a) The urachal remnant forms the median umbilical ligament passing from the apex of the bladder to the umbilicus.
(b) The neck of the bladder rests on the urogenital diaphragm in both sexes.
(c) The distal ureter is posterior to the bifurcation of the common iliac artery.
(d) The bladder is supplied by the superior and inferior vesical artery.
(e) In a plain radiograph, unilateral absence of the perivesical fat stripe is a sign of pelvic pathology.

5. Concerning the bladder:

(a) It is trabeculated except at the trigone.
(b) Colour doppler enables identification of ureteric jets into the bladder.
(c) The wall is of a high signal intensity on T_1- and T_2-W MRI.
(d) It has a normal wall thickness of about 3 cm.
(e) The intramural ureter courses obliquely for about 2 cm before entering the bladder cavity.

6. Concerning the male urethra:

(a) The posterior urethra is divided into the prostatic and spongy parts.
(b) The anterior urethra is divided into the bulbous and penile urethra.
(c) The membranous urethra runs through the external urethral sphincter within the urogenital diaphragm.
(d) The verumontanum is a prominence in the prostatic crest into which the prostatic utricle opens.
(e) The anterior urethra is well visualized on transrectal ultrasound.

7. Regarding the prostate:

(a) The anterior wall of the prostate lies in the arch of the pubis separated from it by retropubic space.
(b) The paired seminal vesicles are separated from the rectum by the peripheral zone of the prostrate gland.
(c) The peripheral zone of the prostate comprises 70% of the glandular tissue.

4.

(a) True – this is extraperitoneal.
(b) False – in the female this is true. In the male, the neck of the bladder rests on the prostate.
(c) False – anterior.
(d) True
(e) True

5.

(a) True
(b) True
(c) False – chemical shift artefact in the frequency-encoding direction produces a high signal within the bladder wall, which may be misleading. On both T_1- and T_2-W MRI the bladder wall is homogeneous and of a low signal intensity.
(d) False – 4–5 mm.
(e) True

6.

(a) False – the prostatic and membranous parts.
(b) True
(c) True – this is 1.5 cm long, and the narrowest, most fixed and least dilatable part of the urethra. Therefore, is most prone to injury during a pelvic fracture.
(d) True
(e) False – the anterior urethra is visualized well by retrograde urethrography. However, the posterior urethra is visualized well by antegrade urethrography when the patient micturates contrast.

7.

(a) True
(b) False – the seminal vesicles are posterior to the prostate and are seprated from the rectum by a dense condensation of the pelvic fascia – Denonvillier's fascia.
(c) True – the glandular tissue has other zones: central zone 25% and transition zone 5%.

(d) The transition zone of the prostate lies at the junction of the central and peripheral zones.

(e) The central zone surrounds the urethra just above the ejaculatory ducts.

8. Regarding the male genital tract:

(a) T_2-W MRI delineates the zonal anatomy of the prostate gland.

(b) Fat suppressed sequences give excellent contrast between the high signal peripheral zone and the periprostatic fat.

(c) The surgical pseudo-capsule is between the enlarged transition zone and the compressed peripheral zone, encountered with increasing age.

(d) The central and peripheral zones are not differentiated on trans-rectal ultrasound (TRUS).

(e) On TRUS the seminal vesicles are very echogenic.

9. Concerning the male genital organs:

(a) The mediastinum of the testis is an incomplete fibrous septum posteriorly.

(b) The vas deferens lies medial to the epididymis.

(c) The testicular artery is a branch of the internal pudendal artery.

(d) The spermatic cord contains the vas deferens, the testicular vessels, cremastric artery and genital branch of genitofemoral nerve.

(e) The testicular vein drains into the pampiniform plexus of veins.

10. Regarding the testis:

(a) The testis has homogeneous medium level echoes on ultrasound.

(b) The mediastinum testis is a posterior and highly echogenic structure.

(c) The epididymis is slightly echopoor compared with the testis.

(d) On T_2-W MRI the testis is either equal to or greater than that of fat.

(e) The pampiniform plexus is of high signal on T_2-W MRI.

(d) False – the narrow transition zone lies just inside the central zone.

(e) True – most carcinomas arise in the peripheral zone, whereas benign prostatic hypertrophy affects the transition zone.

8.

(a) True – the normal peripheral zone has high signal intensity, and the central and transition zones have low intensity.

(b) True

(c) True – changes of benign prostatic hypertrophy. The pseudocapsule and the anatomical capsule are well seen on T_2-W sequences.

(d) False – TRUS shows the central and peripheral zones to be of generally low echogenicity.

(e) False – the seminal vesicles appear as convoluted tubules containing transonic fluid – hence they are of lower echogenicity than the prostate.

9.

(a) True – tunica albuginea is a tough fibrous capsule that forms an incomplete, thickened fibrous septum. Through this run the testicular vessels.

(b) True

(c) False – it arises from the aorta at the level of the renal vessels.

(d) True – and the artery to the vas deferens (from the inferior vesical artery), lymphatics from the testes.

(e) False – the pampiniform plexus of veins above and behind the testis become one single testicular vein as they approach the inguinal ring. The right testicular vein drains into the IVC and the left testicular vein drains into the left renal vein.

10.

(a) True – similar to thyroid.

(b) True

(c) False – echobright and a coarser texture.

(d) True – the fibrous tunica albuginea is of low signal on all sequences. On T_1-W images the testis is of uniformly medium signal less than that of fat.

(e) False – they are seen as signal voids.

11. Concerning the female genital tract:

(a) Lymphatic drainage from the upper third of the vagina is to the internal and external iliac nodes.
(b) The cavity of the uterus is triangular in the sagittal plane.
(c) The retroflexed uterus is better visualized with transabdominal ultrasound than the anteflexed uterus.
(d) In the fetus the cervix is not identified separately from the uterus.
(e) The uterine artery is a direct branch of the aorta.

12. The following are true of the female genital tract:

(a) On T_2-W MRI the junctional zone is a low signal intensity band in the submucosa.
(b) On T_1-W sequences three distinct zones are seen in the uterus.
(c) Normal ovaries are low to medium signal on T_1-W MRI.
(d) After gadolinium DTPA the ovarian follicles exhibit increased signal intensity.
(e) The anatomy of the fallopian tubes are best seen by MRI.

13. Concerning the female genital tract:

(a) Peritoneum covers the superior and lateral aspects of the uterus.
(b) The broad ligaments are formed by the anterior and posterior reflections of peritoneum passing over the fallopian tubes.
(c) The round ligament originates at the lateral angle of the uterus and passes to the labia major.
(d) The internal iliac artery is anterior to the ovary.
(e) Endovaginal ultrasound provides good detail of the adnexal areas.

11.

(a) True – the middle third to the internal iliac and the lower third to the superficial inguinal nodes.
(b) False – cleft in the sagittal plane, triangular in the coronal plane.
(c) False – the opposite is True
(d) False – in fetal life and childhood the cervix is larger than the body of the uterus. By adulthood, the uterine body is twice the size of the cervix.
(e) False – a branch of the internal iliac artery. The ovarian artery is a direct branch of the aorta at L1/2 level.

12.

(a) False – no submucosa exists between the endometrium and myometrium. The junctional zone represents the inner myometrium.
(b) False – on T_1-W sequences the uterus has moderate to low signal intensity. On T_2-W sequences three distinct zones are seen. The endometrium and the cavity appear as a high signal stripe, bordered by a band of low signal junctional zone. The outer myometrium is of medium signal intensity which increases in mid-secretory phase.
(c) True – higher signal on T_2-W MRI.
(d) False – the follicles are low signal foci in surrounding high signal stroma, which enhances after intravenous gadolinium.
(e) False – by hysterosalpingography (HSG).

13.

(a) False – the uterus is covered entirely by peritoneum except below the level of the internal os anteriorly and laterally between the layers of the broad ligament.
(b) True
(c) True – passes through the inguinal canal.
(d) False – posterior to the ovary.
(e) True – and the uterus.

14. Regarding the female genital tract:

(a) On T_2-W MRI the cervix has an inner area of low signal intensity continuous with the junctional zone of the uterus.

(b) The use of oral contraceptives and menstrual cycle change the appearance of the cervix on MRI.

(c) The ampulla of the fallopian tube is the funnel-shaped most lateral part.

(d) In a bicornis bicollis variant of the uterus, there are two separate cervical canals.

(e) Contrast spillage in the peritoneal cavity is a sign of patency of fallopian tubes in a hystero-salpingogram.

14.

(a) True

(b) False – appearances do not change.

(c) False – This is the infundibulum. From lateral to medial are the infundibulum, ampulla – wide tortuous outer part; isthmus – long narrow, just lateral to the uterus; interstitial part – pierces the uterine wall.

(d) True

(e) True – contrast filled tubes with extravasation definitely from the ipsilateral tube is a more reliable sign of tubal patency. Interpretation is rendered difficult when contrast pools in the peritoneal space from the contralateral tube when the ipsilateral tube is blocked.

Obstetric anatomy

A. Doss and A. Sprigg

1. Regarding transabdominal ultrasound of the fetus:

(a) Doppler examinations impart less energy when compared with routine ultrasound.
(b) 18 to 20 weeks of gestation is the optimal time to confirm intrauterine location.
(c) Cardiac activity is seen at 5 weeks' gestational age.
(d) Crown rump length is a useful measurement of gestational age at 10 weeks.
(e) The fetal pole is discernible before cardiac pulsation.

2. Concerning ultrasound of the fetus from 18–20 weeks:

(a) The BPD is measured in the axial plane.
(b) The lateral ventricles are echobright structures.
(c) The medial walls of the lateral ventricles are formed by the septum pellucidum.
(d) The third ventricle is normally visualized.
(e) The cerebellar hemispheres are seen as round echopoor structures with a reflective vermis in the midline.

3. Regarding the fetus:

(a) The vertebra are visible as two ossification centres in the body and one in each lamina.
(b) Failure of fusion between the premaxillary part of the frontonasal prominence and the maxillary prominence gives rise to cleft lip.
(c) The four-chamber view during cardiac ultrasound is the primary screening view for cardiac abnormalities.

Obstetric anatomy

ANSWERS

1.

(a) False – the opposite is true. In general, routine ultrasound is considered completely safe in pregnancy, though examinations should be performed only if clinically indicated and the duration should be kept optimal, particularly when using Doppler.

(b) False – it is the first trimester. During the second and third trimester ultrasound is used to estimate gestational age, to detect structural fetal anomalies, fetal lie and presentation and placental position.

(c) False – cardiac activity is visible at 5 to 6 weeks on transvaginal scanning and at 7 weeks on transabdominal scanning.

(d) True – from 6.5 weeks to 10 weeks. Biparietal diameter (BPD) is valid from 12 weeks up to 24 weeks; femur length from 18 to 20 weeks.

(e) False – cardiac pulsation is visible before any discernible morphology.

2.

(a) True – outer edge of the part of the skull near the transducer to the inner edge of the vault further from the probe is measured.

(b) False – the choroid plexus that fills the lateral ventricles is echobright.

(c) True – this is a double membrane and contains the cavum septum pellucidum which may persist in adult life.

(d) False – seldom seen in the normal fetus.

(e) True – at 18 weeks.

3.

(a) False – one ossification centre in each lamina and one in the body. On ultrasound these are seen as a triangle with the base posterior, in an axial view of the abdomen.

(b) True

(c) True

(d) On ultrasound the lungs become progressively echobright as pregnancy advances.

(e) On ultrasound colonic peristalsis is seen in the second trimester.

4. Concerning the fetal abdomen:

(a) The small intestine becomes increasingly echobright towards the end of pregnancy.

(b) The primitive intestinal loop lies outside the abdominal cavity in the first trimester.

(c) A diagnosis of abdominal wall defect can be made at 10 to 12 weeks.

(d) The umbilical vein runs into the left portal vein.

(e) The abdominal circumference is measured as a parameter for gestational age in the second trimester.

5. Regarding fetal ultrasound:

(a) The femur is strongly reflective at 10 weeks.

(b) The distal femoral epiphyses is seen at 36 weeks.

(c) The beginning of ossification of the proximal epiphysis of the humerus is good evidence of lung maturity.

(d) The diaphysis of ulna and radius extend to the same level at the wrist.

(e) The placenta can be identified as a discrete structure from 12 weeks.

(d)   True – due to developing alveoli. The diaphragm is seen as a smooth echopoor band between the chest and abdomen (in contrast to adults where it is echobright). Breathing movements are evident from early second trimester.

(e)   False – small bowel peristalsis is commonly seen in the third trimester and colonic peristalsis is not seen in utero.

4.

(a)   False – it is more echobright in the second trimester due to meconium, and as the fetus swallows more amniotic fluid in later pregnancy the small intestine becomes less reflective.

(b)   True – the intestine twists counter-clockwise for 270° around the superior mesenteric artery and as a result the caecum comes to lie in the right side of the abdomen.

(c)   False –the physiological umbilical hernia disappears at 14 weeks. Abdominal wall should be intact during the middle trimester.

(d)   True – blood flows from the left portal vein into the right portal vein (which perfuses the liver) and into the ductus venosus.

(e)   True – a transverse section through the fetal liver, with the stomach,spine, the ribs in cross-section, the portal vein equidistant from both sides of the liver.

5.

(a)   True – ossifies at 6 to 12 weeks.

(b)   True – the upper and lower femoral epiphyses appear later in the third trimester. The presence of a distal epiphysis in utero on a plain radiograph at 36 weeks signified maturity of the fetus. This is not practised any more.

(c)   True

(d)   True – important relationship, as many bony anomalies foreshorten the distal radius.

(e)   True

The breast

A. Doss and M. J. Bull

1. The breast:

(a) is a tubulo-acinar type of modified apocrine sweat gland.
(b) has mammary glands which develop from the pectoral portion of the milk line.
(c) has lobes that are epidermal in origin.
(d) has lactiferous ductules, acinar ducts and acini that are lined by a single layer of cuboidal epithelial cells.
(e) has the terminal duct lobular unit (TDLU) which consists of 15–20 lobes drained by a single lactiferous duct.

2. The breast:

(a) lies entirely within the deep fascia of the chest wall.
(b) has the greatest proportion of fibroglandular tissue in the upper outer quadrant which gives rise to the axillary tail.
(c) has fibrous strands of deep fascia that pass through it towards the skin and nipple.
(d) has its main blood supply through the lateral thoracic and internal mammary arteries.
(e) has a venous drainage through the azygos system.

3. In the lymphatic drainage of the breast:

(a) The pectoralis major muscle is the reference for the surgical level of nodes.
(b) This includes intercostal and internal thoracic chains.
(c) Level 1 nodes are inferolateral to the pectoralis muscle.
(d) Level 2 nodes are superomedial to the pectoralis muscle.
(e) Excision of level 3 nodes requires radical surgery.

The breast

1.

(a) True

(b) True – the primitive ectodermal milk line runs from the base of the forelimb to the region of the hindlimb.

(c) True

(d) True – the ducts are lined by columnar cells.

(e) False – 15 to 20 lobes drain by lactiferous ducts onto the nipple. The lobes are divided into lobules. A lobule consists of a group of acini supplied by one terminal duct – the terminal duct lobular unit.

2.

(a) False – within the superficial fascia.

(b) True

(c) False – the suspensory ligaments of Cooper are extensions from the superficial fascia.

(d) True – further supply from the thoraco-acromial and intercostal arteries.

(e) True – venous drainage of the breast includes internal thoracic, axillary, subclavian and azygos veins. The anastomoses between the azygos and vertebral venous plexus are important in the spread of metastatic disease to the spinal column.

3.

(a) False – pectoralis minor is the reference.

(b) True – the majority of lymph drains into the axillary nodes. Some lymph flow drains into the opposite breast and upper abdominal nodes.

(c) True

(d) False – level 2 nodes are deep and level 3 nodes are superomedial to this muscle.

(e) True – with division of pectoralis minor muscle.

4. In the breast:

(a) Epithelial proliferation occurs in the secretory phase of the menstrual cycle.
(b) Marked epithelial proliferation occurs within the TDLU with relative decrease in the surrounding fat and connective tissue during pregnancy.
(c) Contrast between fat and soft tissue is optimized by the use of low energy X-ray spectra.
(d) The 45° mediolateral oblique view is used in the single view screening programmes.
(e) There is a progressive decrease of dense fibroglandular tissue with fatty replacement with increasing age.

5. In mammography:

(a) Fibroglandular tissue appears radiolucent compared with fat.
(b) Normal ducts can usually be seen throughout the breast.
(c) Normal intramammary lymph nodes are usually of calcific density.
(d) The optimal examination should include the pectoralis major.
(e) There is a decreased incidence of malignancy with the P2 and DY patterns described by Wolfe.

6. In the breast:

(a) An accessory nipple (polythelia) is usually just inferior to the normal breast.
(b) Accessory glandular tissue is more common than accessory breasts in the axilla.
(c) Hypoplasia of the breast may be linked with Poland's syndrome.
(d) Calcification of sebaceous glands is pathological.
(e) A skin papilloma appears well circumscribed often with a thin lucent rim (halo) caused by air between skin and the compression plate.

4.

(a) False – epithelial proliferation occurs in the proliferative phase under oestrogens, followed by duct dilatation and differentiation under the influence of progestogens in the secretory phase.

(b) True

(c) True – 17.4 and 19.6 keV are the characteristic peaks from a molybdenum anode.

(d) True – this demonstrates the upper outer quadrant to best effect.

(e) True – provides a comparatively diagnostic mammogram.

5.

(a) False – fat appears radiolucent. Image quality emphasizes contrast and penetration of fibroglandular tissue in order to detect small tumours.

(b) False – normal ducts are thread-like and extremely difficult to visualize unless surrounded by fat or in the retroareolar region.

(c) False – they are of soft tissue density, have a lucent fatty hilum and are situated close to a vascular bundle towards the upper outer quadrant.

(d) True – and include the inframammary fold with the nipple in profile.

(e) False – Wolfe graded the amount and distribution of fibroglandular tissue within a breast into four categories. N1 = normal largely adipose tissue; P1 = adipose breast with parenchymal thickening anteriorly, less than on quarter of the breast volume; P2 as P1 but involving greater than one quarter of the breast volume; DY = generalized increased density of the fibroglandular pattern, without a recognizable ductal or nodular appearance. There is an increased risk of malignancy with the P2 and DY patterns.

6.

(a) True – in 2 to 6% of women there is incomplete regression of the milk line.

(b) True – accessory glandular tissue is more common than accessory breasts in the axilla and is separate from the main breast tissue.

(c) True – underdevelopment of the structures of the chest wall or forelimb is Poland's syndrome. Manifests as increased translucency of the affected hemithorax.

(d) False – fine dense punctate calcification of sebaceous glands seen on tangential projection on to the skin surface is a normal finding.

(e) True

7. In ultrasound of the breast:

(a) A 3–5 MHz probe is ideal.
(b) Intramammary fat lobules are hypoechoic compared with the increased echogenicity of fat in the abdomen.
(c) The fibroglandular tissue is relatively hyperechoic compared with the fatty lobules.
(d) Normal intramammary or axillary lymph nodes are usually ovoid, hypoechoic, with a central echogenic focus representing hilar fat.
(e) Acoustic shadowing is always due to pathology.

8. In imaging modalities of the breast:

(a) The ductogram has virtually been replaced by high frequency ultrasound and cytology.
(b) MRI is limited by motion artefact, noise and suboptimal resolution.
(c) The diagnostic yield of MRI is improved by the use of surface coils and fat suppression.
(d) Excellent inherent contrast between fibroglandular tissue and fat enable MRI to be used as a screening tool.
(e) MRI is contraindicated in patients who have a breast implant.

7.

(a) False – 7.5 MHz probe is usually used.
(b) True – in contradistinction to echobright fatty liver or fatty infiltration of pancreas.
(c) True
(d) True – without increased through transmission of sound which is usually seen in hypoechoic cystic structures.
(e) False – though this is an associated finding with malignancy, it may be caused by fibroglandular tissue or the bright curvilinear bands of Cooper's ligaments.

8.

(a) True
(b) True
(c) True
(d) False – the inherent contrast is excellent. However, MRI is not suitable as a screening investigation.
(e) False – MRI may have a place in the imaging of implants, to differentiate scarring from recurrent malignancy after surgery and to establish extent of tumour.

Module 5

Paediatric anatomy

A. Doss and A. Sprigg

1. Concerning the various differences between paediatric and adult anatomy:

(a) The weight of the neonatal suprarenal gland may be 30% of that of a neonatal kidney.
(b) Gastro-oesophageal and vesico-ureteric reflux are common in neonates.
(c) There is less mediastinal and retroperitoneal fat in children compared with adults.
(d) Neonatal kidneys have a more lobulated contour compared with adults.
(e) The curved diaphragm results in mirror image artefacts during ultrasonography of children.

2. Concerning cranial ultrasonography:

(a) It is performed through the anterior fontanelle during the first year of life.
(b) Axial sections, which correlate with axial sections of computerized tomography, are obtained at the level of the basal cisterns.
(c) The choroid plexuses in the lateral ventricles are echobright.
(d) Pulsating middle cerebral arteries are seen in the Sylvian fissure.
(e) The germinal matrix lines the floor of the lateral ventricles above the heads and bodies of the caudate nuclei.

3. Regarding paediatric ultrasonography:

(a) The quadrigeminal cistern is echopoor in the neonate.
(b) Asymmetry of the ventricles is usually pathological in the neonatal brain.
(c) Incomplete ossification of the posterior spinal arches allows an acoustic window for spinal sonography.

Paediatric anatomy

1.

(a) True – due to a large size in neonates the adrenal can be mistaken for the kidney in renal agenesis.
(b) True – and they may be physiological.
(c) True – on axial CT of the chest in children, it is difficult to assess mediastinal structures due to lack of inherent contrast.
(d) True – due to persistence of fetal lobulation after birth.
(e) True – hence gives a false appearance of a mass in the upper abdomen or lower chest.

2.

(a) True – using a 5 MHz sector probe. Sometimes the posterior fontanelle and sutures may be used with a smaller 'foot print' probe.
(b) True – using the pterion (just above and behind the pinna of the ear) as the acoustic window.
(c) True – Elsewhere the lateral ventricles appear echopoor due to CSF. Intraventricular haemorrhage will also appear echobright.
(d) True
(e) True – very vascular tissue, in the caudothalamic notch, is a site of haemorrhage in the preterm infant. Further tissue may be present in the third and fourth ventricle.

3.

(a) False – contrary to expectations, this CSF-filled space is echobright and the reasons are not fully understood.
(b) False – obliquity of the ultrasound probe and position of the head are commoner than pathology. Asymmetry of ventricles can be seen in up to 40% of premature infants and is less than 20% in term babies.
(c) True – only for several months after birth, especially in the lumbar region.

(d) The spinal cord is echopoor with echobright posterior and anterior walls.
(e) The vertebra appears as echobright blocks separated by echopoor intervertebral discs.

4. Regarding the paediatric chest:

(a) The trachea is less prone to compression in a child than in an adult.
(b) Mediastinal widening in young children may be due to a normal thymus.
(c) The thymus enlarges in illness initially and reduces in size during recovery.
(d) A complete 'white out' on a chest radiograph of a neonate is due to collapse or consolidation.
(e) A posterior impression of the oesophagus can be due to aberrant neck vessels.

5. Regarding ultrasound of the gastrointestinal tract:

(a) The mucosa of the pylorus appears echopoor.
(b) The thickness of the normal pyloric muscle should not exceed 3 mm.
(c) The pancreas is more easily visualized in children through the left lobe of the liver.
(d) The left lobe of the liver extends anterior to the spleen.
(e) Splenunculi occur in 15% of children.

6. Concerning the suprarenal glands:

(a) They lie in the anterior pararenal space.
(b) They lose 80% of their weight in the first 2 to 3 weeks after birth.
(c) The glands have an echobright centre and echopoor rim.
(d) The gland on the right lies between the IVC, right diaphragmatic crus, and the upper pole of the right kidney.
(e) The gland on the left lies lateral to the aorta and left diaphragmatic crus, medial to the spleen and behind the stomach.

(d)   True – a central echobright line is present due to the interface between the central part of the anterior median fissure and myelinated ventral white commissure.

(e)   True

4.

(a)   False – trachea and airways are much narrower, more pliable than in adults and more prone to compression and obstruction. Repeated compression may result in a weak and flaccid trachea (tracheomalacia), which collapses and obstructs during expiration.

(b)   True – on T_1-W MRI, this appears as a lobular intermediate signal structure in the superior mediastinum.

(c)   False – sickness, stress and steroids reduce the size of the thymus initially and the gland regrows during recovery – a common cause of erroneous diagnosis of thymic or mediastinal tumours as a cause of the child's sickness.

(d)   False – on expiration a neonate can almost white out the lungs.

(e)   True

5.

(a)   False – mucosa is echobright and muscle is echopoor.

(b)   False – dimensions vary depending on size of the child. However upper limits in the longitudinal section are as follows: 3 mm thickness of pyloric muscle, and 17 mm in length for the pyloric canal. With measurements above these figures pyloric stenosis has to be suspected.

(c)   True – provides an acoustic window.

(d)   True – trace of free fluid between the left lobe of liver and spleen may give rise to an erroneus diagnosis of laceration of the spleen.

(e)   True

6.

(a)   False – in the upper poles of the kidneys in the perirenal fascia.

(b)   False – 80% of the adrenal gland is fetal cortex and this undergoes haemorrhagic necrosis after birth causing loss of 30% of weight in the first few weeks.

(c)   True – and have limbs.

(d)   True

(e)   True

7. Concerning the renal tract:

(a) Ectopic kidneys retain their reniform shape.
(b) Bilateral renal agenesis is diagnosed on antenatal scans.
(c) In crossed renal ectopia both ureters insert on the same side of the bladder.
(d) A horseshoe kidney usually lies above the level of the inferior mesenteric artery (IMA).
(e) In a duplex kidney the ureter of the lower moiety enters the bladder below to that of the upper moiety.

8. Regarding the urogenital system in chidren:

(a) A narrow track may persist from the trigone of the bladder to the umbilicus.
(b) Cystoscopy is the most reliable method of detecting posterior urethral valves in boys.
(c) In the first year of life about 90% of undescended testes lie within the abdomen and the remainder lie in the inguinal canal.
(d) The medullary pyramids of the neonatal kidney are more hypoechoic than older children.
(e) The female urethra is imaged routinely in the oblique projection.

9. Concerning ultrasonography of the neonatal hip:

(a) The examination is performed using a high frequency linear array probe.
(b) The femoral head is a round structure with fine stippled echoes.
(c) The 'V'-shaped acetabulum has the ischium posteriorly and the pubis anteriorly.
(d) The 'α' angle assesses the depth of the acetabulum.
(e) In the dynamic assessment, the hip is flexed and backward pressure is applied and scanned for evidence of subluxation or dislocation.

10. Regarding paediatric bones and joints:

(a) Bone maturation and development are assessed on a single view of the non-dominant hand and wrist.

7.

(a) False – are not moulded by upper abdominal organs and therefore lose the reniform shape.
(b) True – occurs once in 3300 births and is diagnosed in utero due to the presence of oligohydramnios.
(c) False – ureter of the ectopic kidney crosses the abdomen to enter the correct side of the bladder.
(d) False – it cannot ascend through the abdomen completely as the IMA stops the bridge of renal tissue in the lower abdomen.
(e) False – it enters at the normal orifice: the ureter of the upper moiety enters at an ectopic site lower than the normal orifice.

8.

(a) False – from the 'dome' of the bladder the remnant of the urachus may be visible on cystography. This may give rise to midline cysts between the umbilicus and bladder.
(b) False – micturating cystography.
(c) False – 10 to 20% lie within the abdomen and 80 to 90% lie in the inguinal canal.
(d) True – and larger.
(e) False –the male urethra is imaged in an oblique projection. In the female, congenital abnormalities are rare and the urethra is short. Therefore, it is imaged in the anteroposterior projection.

9.

(a) True.
(b) True – the neonatal hip is largely a cartilagenous structure.
(c) True – echogenic bony cup with a central defect – the triradiate cartilage that separates the two bones.
(d) True – this is the angle between a vertical line along the lateral aspect of the ilium and the line joining the outer and the lowest part of the acetabulum – usually about 60°.
(e) True

10.

(a) True – centred over the head of the third metacarpal, the images may be analysed by two different methods.

(b) The central shaft of a long bone (diaphysis) shows increased uptake of radioisotope compared to the metaphysis.
(c) The epiphysis is the ossified area distal to the physis in a long bone.
(d) An apophysis occurs at the sites of insertion of ligaments and tendons.
(e) On ultrasound of the hips, the beta angle assesses the anteversion of the neck of the femur.

(b) False – the opposite is True
(c) True – the physis or cartilagenous growth plate of long bones separates the metaphysis and epiphysis.
(d) True – an accessory area of ossification, which does not contribute to bone length.
(e) False – assesses the prominence of the labrum. Dysplastic hips have low alpha angles and high beta angles.

Module 6

Neuroradiology

A. Doss and P.D. Griffiths

1. Regarding the imaging methods of the skull and brain:

(a) Skull radiograph is sensitive to cerebral pathology.
(b) Contrast between white and grey matter is superior on MRI compared to CT of the brain.
(c) The contents of the middle and posterior fossa of the brain are better visualized with CT than with MRI.
(d) On T_1-weighted MRI, white matter has lower signal (darker) than grey matter.
(e) On T_2-weighted MRI, grey matter has lower signal than white matter.

2. Regarding MRI of the brain:

(a) Cerebrospinal fluid has high signal on T_1-weighted images.
(b) Cerebrospinal fluid has high signal on T_2-weighted images.
(c) In a proton density MRI sequence, grey matter is hyperintense to white matter.
(d) In CT of the brain the white matter is darker than grey matter.
(e) The fornix and anterior commissure are hypointense on T_2-weighted images.

3. Regarding the technique of brain CT and MR:

(a) The axial plane for CT is usually parallel to a line tangential to the orbital roofs running to the anterior margin of the foramen magnum.
(b) The normal choroid plexus and the pituitary gland enhance on post-contrast CT images.
(c) Mechanism of contrast enhancement of gadolinium DTPA is similar to that of iodinated contrast medium.
(d) Rapidly flowing blood is bright on a T_1-weighted MRI.
(e) Time of flight MR angiography is an invasive procedure.

Neuroradiology

ANSWERS

1.

(a) False – investigation of choice for the detection of fractures, relatively insensitive to cerebral pathology.
(b) True
(c) False – MRI is better. It does not suffer from streak artefacts from bone as seen in CT, which masks soft tissue detail.
(d) False – grey matter has lower signal intensity than white matter.
(e) False – white matter is of lower signal than grey matter.

2.

(a) False – cerebral spinal fluid has low signal on T_1-weighted images.
(b) True
(c) True
(d) True – lipid rich myelin is relatively radiolucent.
(e) True – these are white matter tracts and therefore have low signal on T_2-weighted images.

3.

(a) True – this reduces the radiation to the lens of the eye but increases streak artefact within the middle cranial fossa.
(b) True – other structures to enhance are the cranial arteries, veins, dural venous sinuses and the infundibulum.
(c) False – gadolinium DTPA is not visible on MRI. Gadolinium decreases the T_1 and T_2 of hydrogen in its vicinity. Therefore in a T_1-weighted image there is increased signal which shows up as enhancement.
(d) False – there is flow void and in vessels with rapidly flowing blood the signal remains hypointense even with gadolinium.
(e) False – non-invasive technique.

4. Regarding the skull:

(a) The skull vault develops in membrane.
(b) The occipital bone forms part of the central skull base.
(c) Sutures are between bones of cartilaginous ossification.
(d) Perisutural sclerosis is seen in the neonate.
(e) Sagittal sutural fusion occurs before adolescence.

5. In the skull:

(a) The anterior fontanelle (bregma) is between the frontal and parietal bones at the junction of the sagittal and coronal sutures.
(b) The posterior fontanelle (Lambda) closes around the second month after birth.
(c) Pterion usually closes by 3–4 months.
(d) The periosteum is invested externally and internally.
(e) The endosteum is the outer of the two dural layers.

6. Regarding the skull:

(a) Epicranial aponeurosis (galea aponeurotica) is loosely attached to the skull vault.
(b) The skull vault has a high signal on T_1-weighted MR images.
(c) The diploic veins are found between the two tables of the skull.
(d) Emissary veins traverse the skull vault.
(e) Venous lacunae are close to the midline adjacent to the superior sagittal sinus.

4.

(a) True – skull base develops in cartilage.

(b) True – the occipital, sphenoid and temporal bones form the central skull base. Ethmoid and frontal bones complete the five bones of the skull.

(c) False – they are between bones of membranous ossifications.

(d) False – the skull sutures are smooth in the neonate. Through childhood, interdigitations develop followed by perisutural sclerosis.

(e) False – for practical purposes sutural fusion occurs in adolescence, since only in children does the raised intracranial pressure present with head enlargement.

5.

(a) True – the bregma closes in the second year of life.

(b) True

(c) True

(d) True – both externally (pericranium) and internally (endosteum).

(e) True – this is continuous with the connective tissue at the sutures and fontanelle. Both extradural and subdural haematomas may cross sutures although, in principle at least, this anatomical boundary should prevent the spread of extradural collections.

6.

(a) True – but the skin and subcutaneous tissues of scalp are firmly adherent to the aponeurosis.

(b) False – on MRI the subcutaneous fat is of high signal, superficial to a signal void of the skull vault.

(c) True – the diploic space is between the inner and outer tables of the skull and contains marrow and large valveless thin-walled diploic veins, which are absent at birth. These communicate with meningeal veins, the dural venous sinuses and scalp veins.

(d) True – the emissary veins form a rich craniocerebral anastomosis which provides both a route for the spread of infection across the vault and a collateral path in the event of venous sinus occlusion. This is an indirect sign of venous sinus occlusion.

(e) True – venous lacunae are seen as multiple lucencies on skull radiographs.

7. In the skull:

(a) The frontal bone forms in two halves.
(b) The cribriform plate of ethmoid bone is interposed between the orbital plates of the frontal bone in the midline.
(c) The coronal sutures separate the parietal and frontal bones.
(d) The pterion is a point where the frontal, sphenoid, parietal, temporal bones meet.
(e) Anteriorly the parietal bone articulates with the frontal bone and lesser wing of sphenoid.

8. Regarding the sphenoid bone:

(a) The sphenoid air sinuses in the body of the sphenoid are symmetrical structures.
(b) The anterior clinoid process is part of the greater wing of sphenoid bone.
(c) The posterior clinoid process is part of the lesser wing of sphenoid bone.
(d) The posterior part of the floor of the anterior cranial fossa is formed by the lesser wing of sphenoid.
(e) Part of the middle cranial fossa is formed by the greater wing of sphenoid.

9. In the sphenoid bone:

(a) The dorsum sellae is the anterior boundary of the pituitary fossa.
(b) The dorsum sellae merges laterally with the posterior clinoid process.
(c) The foramina ovale, rotundum and spinosum are in the greater wing.
(d) The greater wing separates the frontal lobe of the brain from the infra temporal fossa below.
(e) Foramen rotundum travels from Meckel's cave to the pterygopalatine fossa.

10. Regarding the foramen of the base of the skull:

(a) Foramen ovale transmits the mandibular division of the fifth nerve.
(b) The foramen spinosum is posterolateral to the foramen ovale.

7.

(a) True – normally fuses at 5 years. The intervening suture is known as the metopic suture which may persist wholly or in part into adult life in 5–10% of individuals.

(b) True – most of the floor of the anterior fossa is contributed by the orbital plates of the frontal bone. The crista galli, to which the falx is attached, ascends vertically from the cribriform plate.

(c) True – the parietal bones on either side are separated by the sagittal suture.

(d) True

(e) False – parietal bone articulates anteriorly with the frontal bone and the greater wing of sphenoid and inferiorly with the temporal bone.

8.

(a) False – they are usually asymmetrical structures.

(b) False – it is part of the lesser wing of sphenoid bone.

(c) False – the pterygoid fossa and posterior clinoid are borne on the superior surface of the body of sphenoid.

(d) True – the posterior border of the lesser wing is the sphenoid ridge, meningiomas of skull base arise in this location.

(e) True

9.

(a) False – this forms the posterior boundary.

(b) True

(c) True

(d) False – it separates the temporal lobe of the brain from the infratemporal fossa below.

(e) True – it transmits the maxillary division of the trigeminal nerve – on coronal CT this foramen is demonstrated inferior to the anterior clinoid processes.

10.

(a) True – on coronal CT, the foramen ovale is inferolateral to the posterior clinoid process.

(b) True – it transmits the middle meningeal artery and vein between the infratemporal and middle cranial fossa.

(c) The vidian or pterygoid canal is inferior to the sphenoid sinus.
(d) The internal carotid artery passes through the foramen lacerum.
(e) Foramen of Vesalius transmits an emissary vein and is medial to the foramen ovale.

11. Regarding the temporal bone:

(a) The squamous part of the temporal bone forms the medial wall of the middle cranial fossa.
(b) The styloid process arises inferiorly from the base of the squamous temporal bones.
(c) The seventh cranial nerve (facial) passes through the stylomastoid foramen.
(d) The mandibular fossa is part of the squamous portion of the temporal bone.
(e) The tympanic portion of the temporal bone is a border of the internal auditory canal.

12. Regarding the skull:

(a) The posterior cranial fossa is the largest of the three cranial fossae.
(b) The basisphenoid synchondrosis (in the clivus) is the articulation between the basioccuput and the base of sphenoid.
(c) In the adult the clivus is hyperintense on T_1-weighted MRI.
(d) The occipital bone has a significant diploic space inferiorly.
(e) The jugular foramen lies between the temporal and occipital bones.

13. Regarding the normal skull radiograph:

(a) Vascular markings are present antenatally.
(b) Vascular markings are radiolucent.
(c) The sphenobregmatic sinus runs on the lesser wing of sphenoid.
(d) Venous impressions on the vault are smaller than those due to arteries.
(e) Arterial impressions are parallel to each other and reduce in calibre after branching.

(c) True – it is medial to the foramen rotundum.
(d) False – this foramen contains cartilage and is traversed only by small veins and nerves. The internal carotid artery crosses its cranial part.
(e) True

11.

(a) False – it forms the lateral wall, separated from the parietal bone by the squamosal suture.
(b) False – from the base of the petrous temporal bone. Calcification of stylohyoid ligament may be seen on a lateral radiograph of cervical spine.
(c) True – the stylomastoid foramen is behind the styloid process.
(d) True
(e) False – it forms part of the external auditory canal.

12.

(a) True – the occipital bone forms most of the walls and floor of the posterior cranial fossa.
(b) True
(c) True – due to replacement of red marrow with fat. In children the clivus is hypointense.
(d) False – typically devoid of a diploic space inferiorly. Therefore the hair on end appearance secondary to marrow hyperplasia seen elsewhere on the skull vault, spares this region.
(e) True

13.

(a) False – they do not develop until the postnatal period and persist through life.
(b) True – have indistinct margins and often branch.
(c) False – this is a sufficiently large vein running along the coronal suture, which gives rise to a prominent vascular impression.
(d) False – venous impressions are larger than those due to arteries.
(e) True

14. The following give rise to lucencies within the skull vault on skull radiographs:

(a) Sutures.
(b) Pineal gland.
(c) Normal thinning of the temporal squame and parietal bone.
(d) Choroid plexus.
(e) The dura.

15. The following give rise to calcifications within the vault on skull radiographs:

(a) Vascular impressions.
(b) Parietal foramina.
(c) Pacchionian depression.
(d) Pneumatization.
(e) Habenular commissure.

16. Regarding the meninges:

(a) The three components are the outer fibrous dura, the avascular arachnoid and the inner vascular pia mater.
(b) The dura and the arachnoid form a free space (subdural) which can be appreciated in normal individuals.
(c) The dura mater has two layers which separate to enclose the dural venous sinuses.
(d) The outer and inner layer of the dura give rise to the falx and tentorium.
(e) The dura does not enhance after intravenous contrast on MR imaging.

17. Regarding the skull:

(a) Wormian bones are small bony elements seen in suture lines and suture junctions.
(b) The basal ganglia and dentate nucleus may show punctate calcification with increasing age.
(c) The interclinoid ligaments stabilize the anterior and posterior clinoid processes.
(d) The pineal gland is anterior to the third ventricle.
(e) The superficial temporal artery grooves the inner table of the temporal and parietal bones.

14.

(a) True
(b) False – gives rise to calcification.
(c) True
(d) False – gives rise to calcification.
(e) False – gives rise to calcification.

15.

(a) False
(b) False
(c) False
(d) False – all the above give rise to lucencies.
(e) True – choroid plexus, petroclinoid and interclinoid ligaments are other causes of calcifications seen on a skull radiograph.

16.

(a) True
(b) False – the dura and arachnoid are applied closely, therefore this is a potential space where haemorrhage or pus may accumulate.
(c) True
(d) False – the inner layer of the dura covers the brain and gives rise to the falx and tentorium. The outer layer of the dura is the periosteum of the inner table of skull.
(e) False – normal dura shows contrast enhancement.

17.

(a) True – these are usually normal variants but may be pathological when multiple in conditions such as cleidocranial dysostosis, osteogenesis imperfecta and hypophosphatasia.
(b) True
(c) False – the interclinoid ligaments are dural calcifications seen in the lateral skull radiograph. They are not described to play a role in the stability of the clinoid processes.
(d) False – posterior to third ventricle. Calcification is seen in 50–70% of adult lateral skull radiographs.
(e) False – it grooves the outer table of the temporal and parietal bones.

18. Regarding the meninges:

(a) The falx cerebri consists of two layers and forms a complete partition between the cerebral hemispheres.

(b) The tentorium cerebelli is attached from the posterior clinoid processes and along the petrous ridges.

(c) The uncus of the hippocampus and the posterior cerebral artery lie below the free edge of tentorium.

(d) The free border of the tentorium cerebelli encloses the cavernous sinus on each side.

(e) The diaphragma sellae is pierced by the pituitary stalk.

19. Regarding meningeal blood supply and innervation:

(a) The main blood supply to the meninges is from the middle meningeal artery.

(b) The accessory meningeal artery may arise from the maxillary or middle meningeal artery.

(c) The middle meningeal artery is subdural in location.

(d) Innervation of the dura is primarily from the trigeminal nerve.

(e) The jugular foramen transmits the ninth, tenth and eleventh cranial nerves.

20. Regarding the normal development of the brain:

(a) The neural tube expands to form the three primary vesicles during the twelfth week of intrauterine development.

(b) Hypodense white matter in a pre-term infant's CT brain usually signifies ischaemia.

(c) Vascular supply of the embryonic brain is similar to that of the adult.

(d) MRI is insensitive to assess the progress of myelination.

(e) Most of the gyri are formed by 18 weeks of gestation.

18.

(a) False – incomplete partition between the cerebral hemispheres, extends from the crista galli to the internal occipital protuberance.
(b) True
(c) False – they lie above the free edge of the tentorium and are at risk of compression against the tentorial edge when there is raised intracranial pressure in the supratentorial compartment (coning).
(d) True – on each side of the pituitary fossa before attaching to the anterior clinoid processes.
(e) True

19.

(a) True – however, there are contributions from the cavernous, carotid, ophthalmic and vertebral arteries.
(b) True – this artery enters the skull through the foramen ovale and supplies the meninges.
(c) False – It is extradural and along with the meningeal veins grooves the inner table of the skull.
(d) True – and also from the lower cranial nerves and the first three cervical segments. This may be the reason for cervical pain in cranial subarachnoid haemorrhage.
(e) True

20.

(a) False – during the fourth week of intrauterine development.
(b) False – due to the relatively high water content, white matter of the normal preterm infant appears hypodense and should not be mistaken for ischaemia.
(c) False – the embryonic brain is exclusively supplied by the internal carotid artery, which may persist in the adult when one of the two posterior cerebral arteries is supplied only through the ipsilateral posterior communicating artery.
(d) False – MRI is used to assess the progress of myelination. T_1-weighted inversion recovery images are particularly sensitive to myelination in the first 6 months. Thereafter T_2-weighted images are used.
(e) False – the brain has more gyri towards term.

21. In the paediatric population:

(a) The entire brainstem is myelinated at <u>birth</u>.
(b) The posterior limb of the internal capsule myelinates before the anterior limb of the internal capsule.
(c) The optic radiation myelinates after 12 months.
(d) The adult pattern of myelination is present on T_1-weighted images after 6 months of age.
(e) On T_2-weighted MRI unmyelinated fibres may be visualized at the age of 4.

22. Regarding the medulla:

(a) It is closed superiorly where it is related to the lower part of the fourth ventricle.
(b) The gracile and cuneate columns are on the ventral surface of the medulla.
(c) The dorsal surface of the medulla becomes the floor of the fourth ventricle below the foramen of Magendie.
(d) The glossopharyngeal (ninth), the vagus (tenth), the spinal accessory (eleventh) and the hypo-glossal (twelfth nerves) arise from the medulla.
(e) On axial MRI the pontomedullary junction is denoted by a broad basilar sulcus.

23. The pons:

(a) is concave on the ventral aspect containing mainly transverse fibres which pass posterolaterally as the middle cerebellar peduncle.
(b) is dominated by the posterolaterally directed middle cerebellar peduncles in the lower aspect.
(c) gives arise to the trigeminal nerve.
(d) gives rise to the abducent nerve.
(e) is posterior to the two roots of the facial (seventh) nerve as they pass from the inferior pontine border laterally in the cerebellopontine angle cistern.

21.

(a) False – the ventral pons is not myelinated.
(b) True – at term the posterior limb is myelinated. At 4 months the anterior limb starts to myelinate.
(c) False – myelinates soon after birth.
(d) True – therefore, T_2-weighted images are used after the first 6 months as they show heterogeneous white matter signal intensity in the first 6 months.
(e) True

22.

(a) False – it is closed inferiorly around the central canal continuous with that of the spinal cord and open superiorly with the lower part of the fourth ventricle.
(b) False – on the ventral surface between the anterior median fissure and the anterolateral sulcus on each side is the pyramid and lateral to this is another elevation, the olive. The gracile and cuneate columns are on the dorsal aspect of the medulla.
(c) False – above the foramen of Magendie the dorsal surface becomes the floor of the fourth ventricle, which opens into the cerebellopontine angle on each side through the foramen of Luschka around the inferior cerebellar peduncle.
(d) True – from above downwards.
(e) True – there is a prominent pontomedullary sulcus on each lateral wall.

23.

(a) False – it has a convex bulbous ventral portion at this level.
(b) True – the cerebellopontine angle is lateral to the middle cerebellar peduncle and limited posteriorly by the flocculi.
(c) True – at this level the superior cerebellar peduncle forms the lateral border of the fourth ventricles.
(d) True – the long intracranial course in an anterolateral direction to bend over the petrous apex takes the abducent nerve through the dura covering the sphenoid bone (Dorello's canal) to enter the cavernous sinus.
(e) True – here they are closely related to the vestibular cochlear nerve.

24. The midbrain:

(a) comprises the dorsal tectum and the paired cerebral peduncles.
(b) contains the cerebral aqueduct of Sylvius.
(c) has the nuclei of the third and fourth cranial nerves.
(d) is surrounded by CSF in the ambient cistern laterally and the quadrigeminal plate cistern posteriorly.
(e) is concerned with auditory reflexes.

25. In the head:

(a) The inferior sagittal sinus is usually identified at catheter angiography.
(b) The great cerebral vein and inferior sagittal sinus form a straight sinus.
(c) The transverse sinus commences at the torcular and lies within the outer margins of the tentorium.
(d) An absent transverse sinus is associated with lack of vascular impression along its course on the skull vault
(e) The spinal root of the accessory nerve passes upwards through the foramen magnum.

26. Regarding the diencephalon.

(a) The structures comprising the diencephalon border the third ventricle.
(b) The calcification of the habenular commissure is anterior to the pineal gland.
(c) The anterior commissure consists of myelinated fibres in the lamina terminalis.
(d) The thalami extend anteriorly as far as the inter-ventricular foramen.
(e) The posterior limb of the internal capsule separates the thalamus from the lentiform nucleus.

27. Regarding the pituitary gland:

(a) The pituitary gland is superior to the suprasellar cistern.

24.

(a) True

(b) True – connects the third and fourth ventricle.

(c) True – third nerve nucleus in the tegmentum, fourth nerve nucleus at the level of the inferior colliculi.

(d) True

(e) True – the tectum is posterior to the cerebral aqueduct and consists of a pair each of the superior colliculi – concerned with visual reflexes and the inferior colliculi – concerned with auditory reflexes.

25.

(a) False – it lies in the free margin of the falx cerebri, seen only rarely in adult angiography but more commonly in children.

(b) True – this lies within the quadrigeminal plate cistern.

(c) True – the right is usually dominant receiving almost the entire output of the superior sagittal sinus.

(d) True – the underdeveloped bony depression of the vault is often helpful to identify this normal variant of the transverse sinus. Moreover, the jugular foramen of the corresponding side is under developed and these features are examined with CT.

(e) True

26.

(a) True – the diencephalon includes the thalamus, hypothalamus, pineal gland and habenula.

(b) True – connects the habenula on each side.

(c) True – this is the anterior limit of the diencephalon. A line joining the anterior and posterior commissures on midline sagittal MR scans (the AC–BC line) is a standard reference in image guided stereotactic surgery.

(d) True

(e) True

27.

(a) False – the suprasellar cistern is a superior relation to the pituitary containing the optic pathways and the Circle of Willis.

(b) The thickness of the infundibulum normally exceeds the diameter of the basilar artery.
(c) The posterior pituitary usually returns a high signal on T_1-weighted images.
(d) Mal-descended pituitary tissue may be found as a soft tissue mass expanding the infundibulum.
(e) The pituitary gland is usually of a constant size in the adult.

28. Regarding the basal ganglia:

(a) They are part of the extra-pyramidal system.
(b) The head of the caudate nucleus indents the anterior horn of the lateral ventricle.
(c) The lentiform nucleus comprises the lateral globus pallidus and the medial putamen.
(d) The claustrum is a thin sheet of white matter between the putamen and insula.
(e) The lentiform nucleus is bounded medially by the internal capsule.

29. Regarding the motor pathways:

(a) The upper motor neurons arise in the pre-central gyrus of the frontal lobe.
(b) The fibres from the primary motor cortex join the corona radiata which converges towards the internal capsule.
(c) The anterior limb of the internal capsule is supplied by the artery of Huebner (from the anterior cerebral artery).
(d) The white matter above the lateral ventricle is known as the corona radiata.
(e) The corticospinal fibres are found in the anterior limb of the internal capsule.

30. Regarding the cerebral hemispheres:

(a) The corpus callosum is the largest of the commissural tracts.
(b) The forceps major are the fibres into the frontal white matter from the corpus callosum.
(c) The central sulcus (Rolandic fissure) separates the frontal and parietal lobes.

(b)   False – the infundibulum is larger in girls, but it should not exceed the diameter of the basilar artery.

(c)   True – this is thought to be due to neural secretory granules in the pituitary.

(d)   True – usually as a rounded high signal mass.

(e)   False – in some individuals it may appear as a thin rim of tissue at the base of the sella (partially empty sella) and in females of child-bearing age the pituitary will fill the sella and have a superior convex margin.

28.

(a)   True – they consist of the caudate and lentiform nuclei, together known as the corpus striatum, the amygdala and claustrum.

(b)   True – the tail of the caudate nucleus comes to lie above the temporal horn and is not readily seen on MRI.

(c)   False – the larger lateral component is the putamen and the smaller medial component is the globus pallidus.

(d)   False – the claustrum is a thin sheet of grey matter.

(e)   True

29.

(a)   True

(b)   True

(c)   True – the anterior choroidal artery supplies the posterior limb and the genu is supplied by the lenticulostriate arteries.

(d)   False – this is the centrum semiovale.

(e)   False – they are found in the posterior limb, corticobulbar fibres are present in the genu.

30.

(a)   True – others are the projection fibres and association fibres.

(b)   False – forceps minor into frontal white matter and forceps major into occipital lobes from the corpus callosum, respectively.

(c)   True

(d) The parieto-occipital fissure runs obliquely on the medial aspect of each hemisphere.
(e) The sylvian or lateral fissure separates the inferior surface of the frontal lobe and the superior surface of the temporal lobe.

31. Regarding the limbic system:

(a) It includes the limbic lobe, olfactory apparatus and the septal areas.
(b) The limbic lobe can be divided into a large limbic gyrus and two slender intra-limbic gyri.
(c) The limbic gyrus includes the subcallosal gyrus and the cingulate gyrus.
(d) The parahippocampal gyrus forms part of the mesial temporal lobe.
(e) The hippocampus lies in the roof of the temporal horn of the lateral ventricles.

32. Regarding the cerebral ventricles:

(a) They contain between 20 and 25 ml of cerebrospinal fluid in the young adult.
(b) The lateral ventricles are roofed by the fibres of the corpus callosum.
(c) Septum pellucidum separates the anterior horns and bodies of the lateral ventricles.
(d) Persistent cavum septum pellucidum is found in approximately 10% of adults.
(e) The cavum vergae is a continuation of the cavum septum pellucidum beneath the splenium.

33. Regarding the ventricles and basal cisterns:

(a) The trigone of the lateral ventricle is the confluence of the body, occipital and temporal horns.
(b) Calcification of the choroid plexus is more common on the lateral skull radiograph than on CT.
(c) The velum interpositum is a cisternal space above the fornix.
(d) The internal cerebral veins are located in the quadrigeminal plate cistern
(e) The cavum vergae extends anterior to the foramen of Monro above the fornix.

(d) True
(e) True

31.

(a) True
(b) True
(c) True
(d) True
(e) False – it lies in the floor of the temporal horn of the lateral ventricles.

32.

(a) True
(b) True – the choroid plexus is invaginated into the medial walls of the lateral ventricles and into the roofs of the third and fourth ventricles through the choroidal fissure.
(c) True – it is a midline triangular sheet attached above and anteriorly to the corpus callosum and posteriorly to the fornix.
(d) True
(e) True

33.

(a) True – the choroid plexuses of the lateral ventricle are here and almost invariably calcify and appear as high attenuation structures on CT.
(b) False
(c) False – a cisternal space below the fornix formed by infolding of the tela choroidea.
(d) False – they are in the cistern of the velum interpositum.
(e) True

34. Regarding the fourth ventricle:

(a) In sagittal section it is triangular with an anterior floor and a roof directed to the apex.
(b) The upper part of the roof is formed by the superior cerebellar peduncles.
(c) The cerebrospinal fluid flows cranially from the fourth to the third ventricles.
(d) CSF flows out into the basal cisterns.
(e) Intraventricular tumours spread through the foramen of Luschka into the subarachnoid spaces.

35. Regarding the subarachnoid cisterns:

(a) The cisterna magna lies between the pons and the postero-inferior surface of the cerebellum.
(b) The cisterna magna is continuous below with the spinal subarachnoid space.
(c) The cisterna magna contains the vertebral, posterior inferior cerebellar arteries through its lateral part.
(d) The basilar artery lies in the pontine cistern.
(e) The ambient cistern surrounds the midbrain and transmits the posterior cerebral and superior cerebellar arteries.

36. Regarding the subarachnoid cisterns:

(a) The chiasmatic or suprasellar cistern contains the circle of Willis.
(b) The chiasmatic cistern leads posteriorly to the interpedencular cistern.
(c) The cistern of the great cerebral vein is the quadrigeminal cistern.
(d) The confluence of the vein of Galen and inferior sagittal sinuses occur in the quadrigeminal cistern.
(e) The pericallosal artery runs in the cistern of the lamina terminalis.

37. Regarding the intracranial circulation:

(a) When present, the trigeminal artery arises from the vertebral artery.
(b) The internal carotid artery is the larger of the two terminal branches of the common carotid artery.

34.

(a) True
(b) True
(c) False – caudally through the third and fourth ventricles.
(d) True
(e) True

35.

(a) False – between the medulla and the postero-inferior surface of the cerebellum.
(b) True – and receives CSF from the fourth ventricle via the foramen of Magendie and Luschka.
(c) True – it also contains the ninth, tenth and eleventh nerves.
(d) True
(e) True – and the basal veins of Rosenthal and the trochlear nerve.

36.

(a) True
(b) True – these contain the terminal basilar artery with branches and the occulomotor nerves. Blood within the cistern may be the only evidence of a subarachnoid haemorrhage.
(c) True – this lies adjacent to the superior surface of the cerebellum and extends superiorly around the splenium of the corpus callosum. It contains the posterior cerebral, posterior choroidal and superior cerebellar arteries and the trochlear nerve.
(d) True
(e) False – it runs in the callosal cistern and the anterior communicating artery runs in the cistern of the lamina terminalis.

37.

(a) False – arises from the internal carotid artery, and represents the embryonic connection between the carotid and basilar arteries which rarely persist into adulthood.
(b) True

(c) The internal carotid enters the cranial cavity via the carotid canal in the petrous bone.

(d) The internal carotid artery enters the subarachnoid space just inferomedial to the posterior clinoid process.

(e) The internal carotid artery terminates into its major branches just medial to the optic chiasm.

38. Regarding the intracranial circulation:

(a) The carotid siphon is the fusiform dilatation at the origin of the common carotid artery.

(b) The ophthalmic artery is the first supraclinoid branch of the internal carotid artery.

(c) The anterior choroidal artery arises distal to the posterior communicating artery.

(d) The internal carotid artery terminates below the anterior perforated substance by dividing into the anterior and middle cerebral arteries.

(e) The T-shape bifurcation into anterior and middle cerebral arteries lies in the direct coronal plane.

39. Regarding the circle of Willis:

(a) It is in the suprasellar cistern.

(b) The circle of Willis is complete in the majority of individuals.

(c) Intracranial cross flow of contrast agent can be tested by manual compression of one cervical carotid artery, while the other is injected with contrast medium.

(d) The pre-communicating (A1) segment of the anterior cerebral artery may be hypoplastic.

(e) The largest of the perforating medial lenticulostriate branches is the Heubner's recurrent artery usually arising from the proximal A2 segment.

40. Regarding the intracranial circulation:

(a) The middle cerebral artery runs laterally through the Sylvian fissure.

(b) The anterior cerebral arteries lie in close proximity to each other in the interhemispheric fissure.

(c) True – it runs approximately horizontally and anteromedially across the upper half of the foramen lacerum, turns upwards and medially to enter the posterior part of the cavernous sinus.
(d) False – inferomedial to the anterior clinoid process.
(e) False – just lateral to the optic chiasm.

38.

(a) False – this is the U-shaped loop formed by the cavernous and immediately supra cavernous portions of the internal carotid artery (contrast to carotid body).
(b) True
(c) True
(d) True
(e) False – this is directed posterolaterally and necessitates an oblique projection to display the tuning fork-like arrangement of the anterior and middle cerebral arteries enface.

39.

(a) True
(b) False
(c) True
(d) True – its distal territory in that case is supplied by the contralateral anterior cerebral artery via the anterior communicating artery.
(e) True – this supplies the anterior limb of the internal capsule and parts of the caudate nucleus and globus pallidus.

40.

(a) True
(b) True

(c) The right and left posterior cerebral arteries are the first branches of the basilar artery.

(d) The thalamostriate arteries are branches of the middle cerebral artery that supply the majority of the thalamus.

(e) The lateral surfaces of the frontal lobes are supplied by the anterior cerebral artery.

41. Regarding the anatomic variants of the intracranial circulation:

(a) The commonest variation of the circle of Willis involves the posterior communicating artery.

(b) The hypoplastic anterior communicating artery may occur in 15–20% of individuals.

(c) Both anterior cerebral vessels may be supplied from one side in 2% of individuals.

(d) The azygos artery runs in the interhemispheric fissure.

(e) The trigeminal artery may arise from the middle meningeal artery to supply the trigeminal and facial ganglia.

42. Regarding the intracranial venous anatomy:

(a) The cortical veins are usually variable.

(b) The superior sagittal sinus is roughly circular in cross-section.

(c) Most of the flow in the superior sagittal sinus is directed to the left transverse sinus.

(d) Valves in the superior sagittal sinus maybe mistaken for thrombus.

(e) The superior sagittal sinus may bifurcate well above its normal termination at the internal occipital protuberance.

(c)   False – the basilar artery terminates by dividing into these.

(d)   False – branches of the posterior cerebral artery.

(e)   False – most of the lateral surfaces of the hemispheres are supplied by the frontal, parietal, angular, superior temporal branches of the middle cerebral arteries from which they arise in the insular.

41.

(a)   True – this vessel may be small in 22%, or may be large and associated with a reduced size of the proximal part of the ipsilateral posterior cerebral arteries and receives its supply from the middle cerebral artery in 15%. This is the fetal posterior communicating artery.

(b)   False – 3%.

(c)   True

(d)   True – the azygos artery is formed when the anterior cerebral arteries fuse approximately to form a single trunk in-between the hemispheres before dividing near the genu of the corpus callosum.

(e)   False – this represents embryonic connections between the carotid and basilar arteries, which rarely persist into adulthood. The trigeminal artery, the commonest of these, arises from the internal carotid artery just before it enters the cavernous sinus and passes lateral to the dorsum sella to the upper basilar artery.

42.

(a)   True

(b)   False – triangular in cross-section – hence a non-enhancing thrombus in this sinus gives the 'empty triangle' or 'empty delta' sign. The sinus usually begins near the crista galli, increases in size from the front backwards; it may not develop anterior to the coronal suture and mimics occlusion in this region.

(c)   False – most of the flow is directed to the right transverse sinus. From the deep venous system blood flows into the left transverse sinus.

(d)   False – the dural sinuses are valveless, trabeculated venous channels. Arachnoid granulations may appear as filling defects and cause confusion.

(e)   True – the intervening space is mistaken for non-enhancing thrombus – false-positive empty triangle or empty delta sign.

43. Regarding the dural venous sinuses:

(a) The sigmoid sinuses are a continuation of the transverse sinuses on each side.
(b) Prominent arachnoid granulations may show up as intraluminal filling defects in the transverse sinus.
(c) Erosive changes in the marginal petrous bone adjacent to the sigmoid sinus may be a normal variant.
(d) An occipital sinus is in the midline running from the foramen magnum towards the torcula.
(e) The intercavernous sinuses are situated on either side of the pituitary fossa.

44. Regarding the cavernous sinus:

(a) It receives the superior and inferior ophthalmic veins.
(b) They communicate with the transverse sinuses via the inferior petrosal sinus on each side.
(c) The internal carotid artery pursues an S-shaped course through the sinus before piercing its dural roof.
(d) The third, fourth and divisions of the fifth cranial nerve run in separate dural tunnels in the lateral wall of the sinus.
(e) The abducent nerve lies inferior to the maxillary nerve in the cavernous sinus.

45. Regarding the venous sinuses:

(a) Meckel's cave is a dural recess anterior to the cavernous sinus.
(b) The sphenoparietal sinus is a medial extension of the Sylvian vein.
(c) The inferior petrosal sinus drains the cavernous sinus into the transverse sinus.
(d) The superior anastomotic vein of Trolard runs from the superficial middle cerebral (Sylvian) vein to the superior sagittal sinus.
(e) The venous angle is where the great cerebral vein joins the inferior sagittal and straight sinuses.

43.

(a)   True
(b)   True – there may be larger 'cavernous nodules' which may be seen as intraluminal filling defects.
(c)   True – this may be due to the pseudoerosive changes, and normal petromastoid aeration is a useful guide to this variant.
(d)   True – the sinus is not usually identified at angiography. At the foramen magnum it anastomoses with the marginal sinuses.
(e)   False – the paired cavernous sinuses are situated in the side of the pituitary fossa and they connect with each other through the intercavernous sinuses.

44.

(a)   True
(b)   False – via the superior petrosal sinus on each side.
(c)   True – the internal carotid artery pierces the dural roof of the cavernous sinus medial to the anterior clinoid process.
(d)   False – they run in a common dural tunnel in the lateral wall of the sinus to reach the superior orbital fissure.
(e)   False – it lies free within the sinus applied to the lateral wall of the internal carotid artery.

45.

(a)   False – this is posterior to the cavernous sinus and is occupied by the trigeminal ganglion.
(b)   True – the Sylvian vein or the superficial middle cerebral vein forms an arc along the surface of the Sylvian fissure and is continuous with the sphenoparietal sinus.
(c)   False – into the jugular bulb which is a focal dilatation of the internal jugular vein at the jugular foramen.
(d)   True – the inferior anastomotic vein of Labbe connects the superficial middle cerebral vein with the transverse sinuses.
(e)   False – the venous angle is the confluence of the thalamostriate and septal veins behind the interventricular foramen of Munro to form the internal cerebral vein.

46. Regarding the vertebrobasilar arterial system:

(a) The most proximal and largest branch of the vertebral artery is the posterior inferior cerebellar artery.
(b) The anterior inferior cerebellar artery arises from the distal end of the vertebral artery.
(c) The superior cerebellar artery is related to the oculomotor nerve.
(d) The pre-communicating (P1) segment of the posterior cerebral artery extends from the basilar bifurcation to the origin of the inferior temporal artery.
(e) The ambient segment (P2) of the posterior cerebral artery courses around the cerebral peduncles above the tentorium.

47. Regarding imaging methods of the eye and orbit:

(a) Soft tissue structures of the orbit are shown well on CT.
(b) The bony orbit and optic canal together with the adjacent osseous structures are best shown by MRI.
(c) The posterior segment of the optic nerve is satisfactorily shown by sonography.
(d) Dacryocystography is usually done with injection of contrast medium into the superior canaliculi.
(e) Fat suppression sequences on MRI are rarely helpful.

48. Regarding the orbit:

(a) Zygoma forms part of the medial wall.
(b) The triangular floor of the orbit is formed only by the orbital process of the maxillary bones.
(c) The inferior orbital fissure separates the floor and the medial wall of the orbit.
(d) The lateral wall of the orbit is formed by the zygomatic bone and more posteriorly by the greater wing of the sphenoid.
(e) The superior wall or roof is formed by the orbital plate of the frontal bone and the lesser wing of the sphenoid.

46.

(a) False – this is the largest and most distal branch.

(b) False – this is a branch of the basilar artery.

(c) True – this is a branch of the basilar artery near to its terminal division and comes to lie inferior to the oculomotor nerve, which separates it from the posterior cerebral artery.

(d) False – the P1 segment extends from the basilar bifurcation to the origin of the posterior communicating artery. The thalamic perforating arteries, which arise from both the P1 segments and the posterior communicating artery, give extensive supply to the thalamus, hypothalamus, the third nerve and the fourth nerve and to the internal capsule.

(e) True – the P2 segment may be compressed against the tentorial edge when there is uncal pressure on the midbrain in the event of raised intracranial pressure. Therefore, infarction of the occipital lobe is a recognized consequence.

47.

(a) True

(b) False – these are best shown by fine section, bone algorithm CT. Plain films may show major fractures. Contents of the optic canal can be shown only by MRI.

(c) False – the anterior part of the optic nerve can be shown by sonography, but CT or MRI is required for demonstration of the posterior segments. MRI reliably shows the internal structure of the non-expanded nerve and sheath.

(d) False – usually the inferior canaliculi.

(e) False

48.

(a) False – the medial wall is formed from front to back by the following: the frontal process of the maxilla, the nasal bone, the lacrimal bone, the orbital plate of the maxilla, the ethmoid bone, the frontal bone, and at the apex the sphenoid bone contributes a small portion.

(b) False – this is formed from medial to lateral by the orbital plate of the maxilla, and the zygomatic bone.

(c) False – this separates the lateral wall from the floor of the orbit.

(d) True

(e) True

49. Regarding the orbit:

(a) The optic canal is formed by the two roots of the lesser wing of the sphenoid bone.
(b) The superior orbital fissure is a triangular slit between the greater and lesser wings of sphenoid.
(c) The medial ends of the inferior and superior orbital fissures are closely related.
(d) The inferior orbital fissure transmits a branch of the maxillary division of the fifth cranial nerve from the middle cranial fossa.
(e) The inferior orbital fissure extends from the middle cranial fossa into the orbit.

50. Regarding the eye:

(a) The lacrimal artery may give rise to a recurrent branch which communicates with the middle meningeal artery.
(b) The intra-orbital segment of the optic nerve is the shortest portion of the nerve.
(c) Fat from the orbit may extend posteriorly into the cavernous sinus.
(d) Direct spread of tumour and infection from the sphenoid sinus to the optic canal may occur.
(e) The blood supply to the optic chiasm is through the basilar artery.

51. Regarding imaging methods of the ear:

(a) High resolution computerised tomography (HRCT) is the examination of choice for the contents of the internal auditory meatus.
(b) HRCT is the technique of choice to look at the anatomy of the petrous temporal bone.
(c) Contrast-enhanced CT is the technique of choice to image the cranial nerves in the cerebellopontine angle cistern.
(d) Tomography should be used to assess the contour of the internal auditory canal.
(e) The whole of the inner ear labyrinth is adequately demonstrated by HRCT.

49.

(a) True
(b) True – this transmits the first division of the fifth and third, fourth and sixth cranial nerves as well as the ophthalmic veins and the branch of the middle meningeal artery.
(c) True
(d) False – it transmits this nerve after it has passed from the middle cranial fossa into the pterygopalatine fossa via the foramen rotundum.
(e) False – the inferior orbital fissure anteriorly forms an opening between the orbital cavity and the infra temporal fossa. More posteriorly it forms an opening between the orbit and the pterygopalatine fossa.

50.

(a) True – this is important because embolization of the middle meningeal artery can endanger the territory of the ophthalmic artery, which gives rise to the lacrimal artery.
(b) False – it is the longest of the four segments, which are intra-ocular, intra-orbital, intracanalicular and intracranial. It measures about 3 cm in length.
(c) True
(d) True – the periosteum of the optic canal may be in direct contact with that of the sphenoid sinus.
(e) False – it is through the anterior cerebral and internal carotid artery. The posterior cerebral artery gives branches to the lateral geniculate body, lower fibres of optic radiation and visual cortex. The middle cerebral artery gives branches to the upper fibres of optic radiations and inconsistently to the occipital poles.

51.

(a) False – MRI is the examination of choice for the contents of the internal auditory meatus and the cerebellopontine angles cistern.
(b) True – MRI gives complementary information of the surrounding soft tissue structures including the facial and auditory nerves.
(c) False – MRI
(d) False – superseded by CT and MRI.
(e) False – the bony labyrinth of the inner ear is demonstrated by HRCT, and the membranous labyrinth is shown by MRI.

52. Regarding the development and anatomy of the ear:

(a) After birth the inner ear continues to grow and attains adult proportions by 2 years of age.
(b) The bony labyrinth of the inner ear is the last structure of the cranium to ossify after birth.
(c) Congenital variants of the middle and inner ear are usually associated.
(d) The lateral two-thirds of the external auditory meatus is cartilaginous.
(e) The tympanic membrane is embedded in the bone of the tympanic ring.

53. Regarding the middle ear and mastoid:

(a) The middle ear is housed in the petrous bone with the tympanic membrane laterally and inner ear medially.
(b) The middle ear is divided into three divisions in the coronal plane.
(c) The aditus ad antrum is a communication from the attic of the middle ear to the middle cranial fossa.
(d) The promontory overlies the basal turn of the cochlea.
(e) The oval window is behind and below the promontory.

54. Regarding the middle ear:

(a) The ossicular chain of malleus, incus and stapes connect the tympanic membrane with the round window.
(b) The head of the malleus and the incudomalleal articulation are situated in the mesotympanum.
(c) The incus lies posterior to the malleus.

52.

(a)   False – the inner ear is essentially of adult size and form at birth.
(b)   False – at birth the bony labyrinth is the only part of the cranium to have ossified fully.
(c)   False – the pinna, external auditory meatus and middle ear appear around the eighth week of gestation and arise from the first and second branchial arches. The inner ear develops with the formation of the optic capsule at about the third week of gestation. Therefore, congenital anomalies of the external ear and middle ear are commonly associated and those of the inner ear are usually isolated.
(d)   False – the lateral one-third is cartilaginous and the medial two-thirds are osseous.
(e)   True – The superior portion of this ring is known as the scutum and is the lateral wall of the epitympanum.

53.

(a)   True
(b)   True – the superior epitympanum or attic is separated by a thin layer of bone called tegmen tympanum from the middle cranial fossa. The mesotympanum and hypotympanum are the middle and inferior divisions which are formed by lines drawn along the superior and inferior margins of external auditory meatus.
(c)   False – this is a communication between the attic and the mastoid air cells and is of importance as middle ear infection may spread to the mastoid air cells, which are related posterior to the sigmoid sinus and cerebellum in the posterior cranial fossa.
(d)   True
(e)   False – the oval window into which the base of the stapes inserts is above and behind the promontory. The round window, which is covered by membrane, is below and behind the promontory.

54.

(a)   False – connect the ossicles with the oval window.
(b)   False – they are in the epitympanic recess.
(c)   True

(d) The incudomalleal and incudostapedial joints have synovial articulation.

(e) The Eustachian tube opens into the inner ear.

55. Regarding the inner ear:

(a) The membranous labyrinth surrounds the bony labyrinth of the inner ear.

(b) The cochlea contains the organ of Corti.

(c) Each semi-circular canal is at about 45° to the other.

(d) The membranous labyrinth is concerned with equilibrium.

(e) The membranous labyrinth is of high signal intensity on T_1-weighted MRI.

56. Regarding the internal auditory meatus:

(a) The anterior wall of the internal auditory canal is shorter than the posterior.

(b) The facial and vestibulocochlear nerves in the internal auditory meatus are best studied using T_1-weighted MRI.

(c) The crista falciformis divides the internal auditory meatus vertically into two compartments.

(d) The lamina cribrosa is at the medial end of the internal auditory meatus.

(e) The facial and vestibulocochlear nerves may form a single bundle as they cross the cerebellopontine angle cistern.

(d) True – they are less prone to those diseases affecting synovial joints elsewhere in the body.
(e) False – the lower part of the middle ear continues inferiorly with the Eustachian tube which opens into the lateral wall of nasal pharynx. This is bony at first and cartilaginous in its lower portion.

55.

(a) False – the bony labyrinth surrounds the membranous labyrinth.
(b) True – concerned with reception of sound.
(c) False – at right angles to the others, and the anterior and posterior canals lie in the vertical plane.
(d) True
(e) False – this contains fluid therefore has high signal intensity on T_2-weighted MRI. The saccule and utricle situated anteriorly and posteriorly within the vestibule cannot be resolved separately by MRI.

56.

(a) False – the opposite is true
(b) False – the meatus contains cerebrospinal fluid, is lined completely with dura and pia-arachnoid and transmits the facial and vestibulocochlear nerves and the labyrinthine artery, which enter its medial opening into the posterior fossa, the porus acousticus. In the majority of cases studied with axial high resolution T_2-weighted MRI the facial nerve can be seen separately anterior to the vestibulocochlear nerve.
(c) False – the internal auditory meatus is divided by the horizontal crista falciformis and vertical crests into four compartments. The facial nerve and the intermediate nerve occupy the anterosuperior quadrant. The cochlear branch of the vestibulocochlear nerve occupies the antero-inferior quadrant. The superior and inferior vestibular branches of the vestibulocochlear nerve are found in the posterior quadrant.
(d) False – the lamina cribrosa is at the lateral end of the internal auditory meatus through which the facial nerve passes to enter the facial canal and the vestibulocochlear nerve which gives branches to the cochlea and vestibule.
(e) True

57. Regarding the facial (seventh) nerve:

(a) The intermediate nerve of the facial nerve is the large motor root.
(b) The first labyrinthine segment of the facial nerve extends anteromedially from the internal auditory meatus.
(c) The greater superficial petrosal nerve arises from the geniculate ganglion.
(d) The first genu of the facial nerve is directed posteriorly from the geniculate ganglion.
(e) The mastoid segment is a continuation from the second genu of the facial nerve.

58. Regarding the cerebellopontine angle cistern:

(a) The flocculus of the cerebellum forms the anterior boundary.
(b) The facial and vestibulocochlear nerves lie here.
(c) It is roughly triangular in shape in the axial plane.
(d) The labyrinthine artery may enter the internal auditory meatus.
(e) The anterior inferior cerebellar artery forms a meatal loop.

57.

(a) False – the facial nerve has a large motor and a small sensory root which is the intermediate nerve. This is too small to be identified either by cisternography or MRI.

(b) False – the first segment of the facial nerve extends anterolaterally from the internal auditory meatus.

(c) True – it carries secretomotor fibres to the lacrimal gland and takes fibres to the palate.

(d) True – the tympanic segment passes along the medial wall of the tympanic cavity beneath the lateral semi-circular canal. Therefore, this part of the facial nerve is vulnerable to inflammatory disease of the middle ear. Coronal CT through the cochlea shows the facial canal twice to produce 'snake's eyes' appearance of the facial nerve above the cochlea.

(e) True – the mastoid segment is directed inferiorly, and the nerve emerges from the skull base through the styloid foramen. This nerve transmits taste fibres from the anterior two-thirds of the tongue to the lingual nerve and the motor fibres to the submandibular and sublingual gland.

58.

(a) False – the cerebellopontine angle cistern is bounded by the posterior surface of the petrous bone laterally, the pons medially and the flocculus of the cerebellum posteriorly.

(b) True – the flocculus lies closely to the anterior/inferior cerebellar artery and may become hyperdense in comparison with the remainder of the cerebellum. This should not be mistaken for an acoustic neurinoma.

(c) True – the other structures in this cistern are the seventh, eighth cranial nerves, the anterior/inferior cerebellar artery and the trigeminal nerve.

(d) True – the labyrinthine artery arises from the meatal loop of the anterior inferior cerebellar artery. On contrast-enhanced CT this may be mistaken for an acoustic neurinoma.

(e) True.

59. Regarding surface anatomy:

(a) The nasion overlies the suture between the frontal and ethmoid bones.
(b) A line joining the parietal eminence on each side forms the smallest transverse diameter of the skull.
(c) The inion is the point lateral to the tip of the external occipital protuberance.
(d) The lambda represents the posterior fontanelle in the newborn and is at the junction of the sagittal and lambdoid sutures.
(e) The coronoid process of the mandible can be felt in front of the tragus.

60. Regarding the anatomy of the head and neck:

(a) The parotid duct can be rolled across the anterior border of the masseter muscle just below the zygomatic bone, with teeth clenched.
(b) The orifice of the parotid duct can be seen within the mouth at the level of the second upper premolar tooth.
(c) The mental foramen is found at the level of the two premolar teeth.
(d) The mental branch of the inferior alveolar nerve emerges from the mental foramen.
(e) The sternocleidomastoid has two heads at insertion.

61. Concerning vertebral levels:

(a) Atlas and dens of axis lie in the horizontal plane of the open mouth in an AP projection.
(b) The hyoid bone lies at the level of the fifth cervical vertebra.
(c) The lower border of the cricoid cartilage is at the level of the sixth cervical vertebra.
(d) The upper border of the thyroid lamina is at the level of the fourth cervical vertebra.
(e) The junction of the pharynx and the oesophagus is at the level of the sixth cervical vertebra.

59.

(a) False – the nasion overlies the suture between the frontal and nasal bones.
(b) False – the line joining each parietal eminence forms the greatest transverse diameter of the skull.
(c) False – the inion is the point on the tip of the external occipital protruberance in the midline.
(d) True
(e) False – the condyloid process lies in front of the tragus and moves forwards and downwards if the mouth is opened. The coronoid process can be identified by placing a finger in the angle between the zygomatic arch and the masseter muscle.

60.

(a) True
(b) False – the orifice of the parotid duct can be seen opposite the upper second molar tooth.
(c) True – the mental foramen is midway between the upper and lower borders of the body of the mandible at the level of the interval between the two premolar teeth.
(d) True
(e) True

61.

(a) True
(b) False – third cervical vertebra
(c) True
(d) True – the common carotid artery bifurcates at this level
(e) True – at this level is the junction of the larynx with the trachea. Also, the vertebral artery usually passes into the foramen transversarium of the cervical vertebra.

Extracranial head and neck (including eyes, ENT and dental)*

A. Doss and M.J. Bull

1. Regarding the head and neck:

(a) The tongue receives innervation from nerves of the first, second, third and fourth pharyngeal arches.
(b) The thyroid gland originates at the apex of the foramen caecum on the developing tongue.
(c) In the Water's view (occipitomental) the petrous ridges should be projected just above the maxillary antra.
(d) Dolan's three lines are useful to identify facial symmetry in the Cauldwell (occiptofrontal) view.
(e) The lateral pterygoid muscle lies inferior and lateral to the medial pterygoid.

2. Regarding the head and neck:

(a) The pterygomaxillary fissure opens into the infratemporal fossa through the pterygopalatine fossa.
(b) The infratemporal fossa communicates with the nasal cavity through the sphenopalatine foramen.
(c) The foramen rotundum opens into the posterior wall of the infratemporal fossa.
(d) The mandibular nerve emerges from the foramen ovale.
(e) The infratemporal fossa is inferior to the lesser wing of sphenoid.

3. Regarding the mandible and the temporomandibular joint:

(a) Each half of the body of the mandible is fixed anteriorly in the midline at the mental symphysis.
(b) The inferior alveolar nerve enters the mandibular canal through the mandibular foramen.

---

* From *Applied Radiological Anatomy.* 'Extracranial head and neck'.

Extracranial head and neck (including eyes, ENT and dental)*

ANSWERS

1.

(a) True
(b) True
(c) False – just below the maxillary antra.
(d) False – in the Water's view.
(e) False – bulk of lateral pterygoid is cranial to the medial pterygoid. Therefore, on axial images the lateral and medial pterygoid appear to be at the same level.

2.

(a) False – the lateral opening of the pterygopalatine fossa into the infratemporal fossa is the pterygomaxillary fissure.
(b) False – the pterygopalatine fossa opens into the nasal cavity through the sphenopalatine foramen.
(c) False – it opens into the posterior wall of the pterygopalatine fossa and transmits the maxillary nerve.
(d) True
(e) False – inferior to greater wing of sphenoid and behind the maxilla.

3.

(a) True
(b) True – enters on the inner surface of the ramus and emerges on the outer surface through the mental foramen

---

* From *Applied Radiological Anatomy.* 'Extracranial head and neck'.

(c) The TMJ has a fibrous articular disc, which separates the mandibular fossa of the temporal bone into lateral and medial compartments.
(d) The disc and the condyle move forward when the mouth is opened.
(e) Arthrography is usually performed in only the inferior compartment.

4. In the nose:

(a) The hiatus semilunaris is situated beneath the ethmoid bulla in the middle meatus.
(b) The sphenopalatine foramina lie behind the superior meatus.
(c) The nasal mucosa is usually symmetrical on MRI.
(d) The main blood supply to the nasal cavity is from the sphenopalatine branch of the maxillary artery.
(e) Little's area is the antero-inferior aspect of the nasal septum.

5. Regarding the paranasal sinuses:

(a) The frontal sinuses are present at birth.
(b) Hypoplasia of maxillary sinus may be seen in up to 10% of normal population, and is seen as high density on plain radiographs.
(c) The ostiomeatal complex is the final common pathway for drainage of secretions from the maxillary, frontal and anterior and middle ethmoid sinuses into the middle meatus.
(d) The greater and lesser wings of sphenoid usually pneumatize.
(e) The anterior midline septum of the sphenoid sinus may be deviated to one side posteriorly.

6. Regarding the salivary glands:

(a) The parotid gland lies beneath the ramus of the mandible.
(b) The parotid gland typically has an attenuation similar to that of muscle on CT.
(c) Stenson's duct runs deep to the masseter muscle.
(d) The submandibular gland has a similar attenuation to the parotid on CT.
(e) The digastric muscle divides the submandibular gland into superficial and deep portions.

(c) False – divides into larger inferior and smaller superior compartments, which do not communicate and function as separate joints.
(d) True – the bilaminar zone – a loose posterior attachment of the condyle to the temporal bone permits this forward translation.
(e) True – this is done for joint function, to diagnose joint perforation and anterior dislocation. More recently, MRI is the technique of choice.

4.

(a) True – ethmoid, maxillary and frontal sinuses drain into the hiatus.
(b) True – serves as a conduit for infection or neoplasm to spread into the orbit or cranial cavity.
(c) False – periodic vascular engorgement results in opening and closing of alternate sides of the nasal airway every 2–3 hours.
(d) True
(e) True – the rich blood supply of the nasal cavity derives from both internal and external carotid systems. The anterior ethmoidal branches of the ophthalmic artery joins the anastomotic network in the nasal septum. Little's area is the most common site of epistaxis.

5.

(a) False – traces of sphenoid and maxillary sinus are present in the neonate. All other sinuses become evident at about 7 or 8 years.
(b) True – not to be confusd with inflammation when seen on a plain radiograph.
(c) True
(d) False
(e) True – its identification is important prior to trans-sphenoidal surgery.

6.

(a) False – lies over the ramus of the mandible and masseter muscle.
(b) False – the attenuation is between fat and muscle.
(c) False – runs superficial to the masseter and turns medially, pierces the buccinator to open opposite the second upper molar tooth.
(d) False – higher than that of parotid gland.
(e) False – mylohyoid divides the gland into superficial and deep portions. The digastric muscle divides the gland into its anterior and posterior portions.

7. Regarding the pharynx:

(a) It extends from the base of the tongue to the level of C6.
(b) The pharyngobasilar fascia at the level of the nasopharynx is deficient as the sinus of Morgagni.
(c) On axial CT and MRI the fossa of Rosenmuller is lateral to the torus tubarius.
(d) The palatine tonsils are between the palatoglossal and palatopharyngeal folds.
(e) The tonsils and adenoids have a high signal on T_2-W MRI.

8. Regarding the larynx:

(a) The epiglottis arises from the cricoid cartilage.
(b) The piriform fossa lies between the aryepiglottic fold and the thyroid cartilage.
(c) The arytenoid cartilage alters the tension of the vocal cords and the shape of the glottis.
(d) The paraglottic space terminates below the cricoid cartilage.
(e) The pre-epiglottic space lies between the base of the tongue and the epiglottis.

9. Regarding the fascial layers of the neck:

(a) The superficial cervical fascia is subcutaneous and extends into the thorax inferiorly.
(b) The superfical or investing layer of the deep cervical fascia envelopes the parotid and submandibular gland.
(c) The middle or visceral layer of the deep cervical fascia lies deep to the strap muscles of the neck.
(d) The deep or prevertebral layer surrounds the brachial plexus.
(e) The carotid sheath receives contribution from only the middle layer of the deep cervical fascia.

10. The parapharyngeal space:

(a) appears hyperintense on T_1-W MRI.
(b) is one of the commonest sites for primary pharyngeal tumours

7.

(a) False – from the base of the skull to the lower border of the cricoid cartilage at the level of C6, where it becomes continuous with the oesophagus.
(b) True – this serves as a potential conduit for neoplastic or inflammatory process to reach the skull base.
(c) False – the fossa of Rosenmuller (the site of origin of up to 50% of nasopharyngeal carcinomas) is posterior and medial to the opening of the auditory tube.
(d) True
(e) True

8.

(a) False – from the thyroid cartilage.
(b) True
(c) True – the cricoid cartilage articulates with the thyroid and arytenoid through synovial joints. Therefore, these joints are susceptible to systemic arthropathies such as rheumatoid disease.
(d) False – the paraglottic spaces lie deep to the false and true cords. They contain fat and terminate at the upper border of the cricoid cartilage. Therefore there is no soft tissue within the cricoid ring.
(e) False – between the epiglottis and hyoid bone.

9.

(a) True – and completely encircles the head and neck.
(b) True – and extends to clavicles, sternum and scapulae.
(c) True – invests the trachea, oesophagus and surrounds the thyroid gland.
(d) True – and the vertebrae, paraspinal muscles. It extends from the skull base to the superior mediastinum.
(e) False – from all three layers of the deep cervical fascia.

10.

(a) True – 'high-signal fatty triangle'.
(b) False – it is characteristically infiltrated, displaced by surrounding masses.

(c) contains the maxillary artery.

(d) is bounded anteriorly by the buccinator space.

(e) is bounded medially by the parotid space.

11. Regarding the thyroid and parathyroid glands:

(a) The pyramidal lobe extends superiorly from the left lobe.

(b) The left lobe is usually larger than the right.

(c) The follicular nature of the thyroid is resolved by high frequency ultrasonographic examination.

(d) ^{99m}Tc pertechnetate imaging provides functional data on the thyroid gland.

(e) The thyroid derives its blood supply from the external and internal carotid systems.

12. Regarding the external carotid artery and its branches:

(a) The ascending pharyngeal artery ascends between the internal and external carotid artery on the posterolateral wall of the pharynx.

(b) The first branch is the lingual artery.

(c) The facial artery contributes to connections between the external carotid and internal carotid arteries.

(d) The occipital artery anastomoses with branches of the vertebral artery.

(e) The superficial temporal and posterior auricular arteries are the two terminal branches of the external carotid artery.

(c) True – and the ascending pharyngeal artery, pharyngeal venous plexuses, mandibular nerve branches and fat.

(d) False

(e) False – laterally by the parotid space, posteriorly by the carotid sheath, medially by the pharyngeal mucosal space, anteriorly by the masticator space.

11.

(a) False – extends from the isthmus in the midline in 40% of subjects.

(b) False – the opposite is true. The right lobe is more vascular than the left and tends to enlarge more in diffuse disorders.

(c) False – the thyroid appears relatively homogeneous in texture and relatively hyperechoic to the superficial sternocleidomastoid muscles.

(d) False – ^{99m}Tc is not metabolized in the thyroid. However, ^{123}I is both trapped and organified, and functional data can be obtained. ^{99m}Tc provides morphological information and will reveal the presence of ectopic thyroid tissue.

(e) False – the paired superior thyroid and inferior thyroid arteries are from the external carotid and thyrocervical trunk (subclavian artery) respectively. The thyroidea ima is an occasional branch of the brachiocephalic trunk on the aortic arch, which supplies the inferior portion of the right lower lobe.

12.

(a) True – an important artery in interventional radiology, it participates in extensive anastomoses with other branches of the external carotid artery, cavernous branches of the internal carotid artery and meningeal branches of the vertebral artery.

(b) False – superior thyroid artery is the first branch.

(c) True – anastomoses with branches of the ophthalmic artery (branch of the internal carotid artery).

(d) True – also sends meningeal branches to the dura of the posterior fossa.

(e) False – superficial temporal and maxillary arteries.

13. Regarding the maxillary artery and its branches:

(a) The maxillary artery passes anteriorly from the parotid gland through the infratemporal fossa.
(b) The maxillary artery lies deep to the temporalis muscle.
(c) The middle meningeal artery enters the anterior cranial fossa.
(d) The superficial temporal artery is usually a straight structure.
(e) The anterior deep temporal artery is a branch of the second part of the maxillary artery.

14. Regarding ultrasonography of the carotid arteries:

(a) In a B-mode study, the wall of the normal carotid artery produces two parallel echopoor layers with a hyperechoic strip between them.
(b) The Doppler flow study measures the velocity of blood flowing through the arteries.
(c) The common carotid arterial Doppler trace resembles that of the external carotid artery.
(d) The internal carotid artery supplies a high resistance circulation.
(e) Flow reversal at the bulb of the bifurcation of the common carotid artery is a normal feature.

15. Regarding venous drainage of the head and neck:

(a) The retromandibular vein drains into the external jugular vein.
(b) The facial veins communicate with the cavernous sinus through the ophthalmic veins.
(c) The external jugular vein drains into the internal jugular vein.
(d) The retromandibular vein is joined by the occipital vein to form the external jugular vein.
(e) The internal jugular vein has no valves.

13.

(a) True

(b) True – 15 terminal branches are given off anterior to the pterygopalatine ganglion.

(c) False – enters the middle cranial fossa through the foramen spinosum. The anterior division is prone to damage in fractures of the skull, giving rise to an extradural haematoma.

(d) False – this artery has a 'corkscrew' appearance compared with the relatively straight branches of the maxillary artery, which enables its easy identification on a lateral angiogram.

(e) True – the branches from the second part of the maxillary artery supply muscles of mastication. The anterior deep temporal artery anastomoses with orbital vessels forming another potential external to internal carotid arterial connection.

14.

(a) False – it produces two parallel echoes, which represent the intima and adventitia with the intervening echopoor layer of the media.

(b) True – and also provides information on direction and flow characteristics.

(c) False – 70% of common carotid arterial blood flow is directed towards the brain. Therefore the common carotid arterial Doppler resembles that of the internal carotid artery.

(d) False – it supplies a capacitance circulation with low total peripheral resistance.

(e) True

15.

(a) True

(b) True

(c) False – drains into the subclavian vein.

(d) False – retromandibular vein is joined by the posterior auricular vein to form the external jugular vein. The occipital vein drains into the internal jugular vein.

(e) False – it has valves just above the inferior bulb, which may prove difficult to pass with a guidewire.

16. Regarding the brachial plexus:

(a) It is formed from the anterior rami of the fifth cervical to the first thoracic nerve roots.
(b) The upper trunk lies between the scalenus anterior and medius muscles.
(c) The middle trunk lies beneath the scalenus anterior muscle.
(d) The five nerve roots eventually give rise to five nerves.
(e) The cords of the brachial plexus form above and behind the pectoralis minor muscle.

16.

(a) True – the fourth cervical and second thoracic roots may also contribute.
(b) True – it is formed by the fifth and sixth cervical roots.
(c) False – the middle trunk is formed by the seventh cervical root. The eighth
     cervical and first thoracic roots unite behind scalenus anterior to form the
     lower trunk.
(d) True
(e) True – and surround the axillary artery, run between the clavicle and first rib to
     enter the axilla, where they divide into their terminal branches.

The vertebral column*

A. Doss and M. J. Bull

1. Regarding imaging of the spine:

(a) The attenuation of fat is higher than that of cerebrospinal fluid on computerized tomography.
(b) Following administration of intravenous iodinated contrast medium, the spinal cord and nerve roots enhance.
(c) Bone and soft tissue is visualized using a window level of 40 HU and a width of 300 HU.
(d) CT myelography shows changes in spinal cord substance.
(e) On T_2-W sequence CSF is of higher signal than neural structures and ligaments.

2. Concerning the vertebral column and the vertebra:

(a) Cervical and lumbar lordoses are primary curves present at birth.
(b) The posterior column is formed by the posterior longitudinal ligament and the neural arch.
(c) The pedicles fuse laterally to form the spinous processes.
(d) Transverse process arises from the lateral aspect of the vertebral bodies.
(e) The pars interarticularis is the part of the lamina between the superior and inferior articular facets.

---

* From *Applied Radiological Anatomy*. 'The vertebral and spinal column'.

The vertebral column*

ANSWERS

1.

(a) False – CSF and water have an attenuation of about zero Hounsfield units – fat is radiolucent and has a lower attenuation of about -60 to -100 and appears darker than CSF.

(b) False – following contrast, the spinal cord, nerve roots and intervertebral discs do not enhance. The spinal meninges, dorsal root ganglia and blood vessels enhance.

(c) False – separate window settings are required to visualize bone and soft tissue as follows: Bone (level 200 HU and width of 1500 HU); Soft tissue (level 40 HU and width 300 HU).

(d) False – shows any alteration in contour. MRI shows changes in spinal cord substance.

(e) True – T_2-W images have a myelographic effect.

2.

(a) False – the thoracic and pelvic kyphoses are primary curves present in fetal life. The cervical and lumbar lordoses are secondary which develop after birth.

(b) False – the vertebral column is a three-column structure. Anterior – anterior longitudinal ligament, anterior annulus fibrosus and anterior part of the vertebral body; middle – posterior longitudinal ligament and posterior annulus fibrosus on each side; posterior – neural arch and posterior longitudinal ligamentous complex including the interspinuos ligament.

(c) False – the posterior neural arch contains laterally the pedicles on each side. The laminae are posterior and fuse to form the spinous process.

(d) False – from the junction of the pedicle and the lamina. The articular processes project superiorly and inferiorly from the junction of the pedicle and lamina.

(e) True – a pars defect is a spondylolysis, which may cause spondylolisthesis of the vertebral body.

---

* From *Applied Radiological Anatomy*: 'The vertebral and spinal column'.

3. Regarding the intervertebral disc:

(a) The intervertebral disc forms a secondary cartilaginous joint between adjacent vertebrae.
(b) The posterolateral portion of the disc is not reinforced by the posterior longitudinal ligament.
(c) The nucleus pulposus is a gelatinous structure containing type II collagen.
(d) The annulus fibrosus has internal and external components which insert into the hyaline cartilage and around the cartilaginous plate beyond the vertebral margins, respectively.
(e) The disc is vascular throughout adult life.

4. In the spine:

(a) The internuclear cleft develops during fetal life to differentiate into the central nucleus pulposus and the peripheral annulus fibrosus.
(b) The cortical compact bone is the weight-bearing component of the body of the vertebra.
(c) The red marrow of children appears hyperintense on T_1-W MRI sequences compared with yellow marrow.
(d) The external annulus is hypointense on both T_1- and T_2-W MRI sequences.
(e) The internuclear cleft is seen as a hypointense transverse band across the mid-portion of the disc on MRI.

5. Concerning ligaments of the vertebral column:

(a) The anterior longitudinal ligament extends from the basiocciput to the anterior surface of the upper sacrum.
(b) The posterior longitudinal ligament extends from the axis to the sacrum.
(c) The anterior longitudinal ligament is more firmly attached to the intervertebral disc than to the vertebral bodies.
(d) The supraspinous ligament joins the tips of adjacent spinous processes from C1 to the sacrum.
(e) The ligamentum flavum is elastic and has a slightly higher intensity on T_1-W MRI compared to the other spinal ligaments.

3.

(a) True – joint surfaces are lined by hyaline cartilage with an intervening fibrocartilage disc.
(b) True – hence many lumbar disc prolapses arise from this region.
(c) True – a remnant of the notochord, it contains up to 90% water and acts as a shock absorber. With increasing age, the disc undergoes progressive dehydration with loss of height and is replaced by fibrocartilage by 80 years of age.
(d) True – the external annulus has thick fibres containing 'type I' collagen similar to fibrocartilage.
(e) False – the rich blood supply to the discs present in infants and children decreases after puberty. By the age of 20 the normal disc is avascular.

4.

(a) False – in the second or third decade an internuclear cleft develops, which represents compacted collagenous fibres oriented transversely, due to invagination of the inner annular lamellae.
(b) False – the vertebral body consists of a mass of cancellous bone surrounded by a cortical rim of compact bone. The cancellous bone has vertical (weight-bearing) and horizontal trabeculae.
(c) False – the red marrow of children appears relatively hypointense on T_1-W sequences. Following intravenous gadolinium, it enhances on T_1-W sequences.
(d) True
(e) True

5.

(a) True
(b) True – above the axis it continues as the tectorial membrane.
(c) False – the posterior longitudinal ligament is firmly attached to the discs and is separated from the vertebral bodies by the emerging basivertebral vein and epidural venous plexuses. The anterior longitudinal ligament is attached firmly to the vertebral bodies and less firmly to the discs.
(d) False – it extends from C7 to the sacrum. Above C7 it continues as ligamentum nuchae and inserts into the external occipital protuberance.
(e) True – it can extend by up to 35% of its length on flexion.

6. In the spine:

(a) The facet joints are synovial joints.
(b) The facet joints are the largest in the lowest two lumbar vertebrae.
(c) The cervical intervertebral foramen is orientated laterally.
(d) The inferior articular process of the vertebra above is anterior to the superior articular process of the vertebra below.
(e) The cervical vertebral bodies are supplied by segmental branches from the aorta.

7. Regarding vertebral venous plexuses:

(a) The internal venous plexus runs in the body of the vertebra.
(b) The external plexus consists of the anterior and posterior compartments.
(c) The internal venous plexus communicates through the foramen magnum with occipital and basilar sinuses.
(d) In the cervical region the external venous plexus communicates freely with occipital and deep cervical vein.
(e) On MRI the course of the basivertebral vein is seen as a signal void.

8. Regarding the vertebrae:

(a) The ossification centres appear at the eighth week of gestation.
(b) The vertebral column ossifies in hyaline cartilage.
(c) There are three primary ossification centres for a typical vertebra.

6.

(a)   True – the intervertebral discs are symphyses; between the laminae, transverse
       and spinous processes are fibrous joints (syndesmoses).
(b)   True – this is where the maximum weight is borne by the vertebral column.
(c)   False – orientated anterolaterally at 45° to the sagittal plane and is thus
       demonstrated using an oblique radiographic projection. In the thoracic and
       lumbar regions they are orientated laterally, and lateral radiographs are
       appropriate to demonstrate them.
(d)   False – the inferior articular process of the vertebra above is posterior to the
       superior articular process of the vertebra below. On axial section at the level of
       the facet joint the superior articular facet is anterior to the joint.
(e)   False – the atlas and axis vertebrae are supplied by the ascending pharyngeal
       and occipital arteries. The other cervical vertebrae are supplied by segmental
       branches from the costocervical, thyrocervical trunks and vertebral arteries.
       The thoracic and lumbar parts of the vertebral column are supplied by
       segmental aortic branches.

7.

(a)   False – this is a plexus of thin-walled, valveless veins in the vertebral canal that
       surrounds the dura mater of the spinal cord and the posterior longitudinal
       ligament. The basivertebral vein runs in the body of the vertebra and drains into
       the internal plexus.
(b)   True – anterior to the vertebral bodies and posterior to the spinous processes,
       respectively.
(c)   True
(d)   True
(e)   False – due to slow venous flow and perivenous fat, the course of the vein is
       shown as high signal.

8.

(a)   True
(b)   True
(c)   True – one in the centrum; one for each half of the neural arch. There are two
       ossification centres in the centrum, which fuse. Failure of one-half of this
       ossification centre to develop results in a hemivertebra.

(d) The neurocentral joints (synchondroses) between the centrum and each half of the neural arch fuse by 7 years of age.

(e) Failure of fusion of the neural arches with the centrum results in spina bifida.

9. Concerning the craniovertebral junction:

(a) The atlas has no vertebral body.

(b) The arcuate foramen is a defect in the posterior arch of the atlas.

(c) The atlas is the strongest of the cervical vertebrae.

(d) The dens of the axis develops entirely from two primary ossification centres.

(e) The dens has more compact bone than the body of the axis.

10. Concerning the craniovertebral junction:

(a) A separation of up to 5 mm in the alignment of the lateral borders of the lateral masses of the atlas and axis vertebra in adults is acceptable.

(b) Disruption of Harris' ring indicates a fracture on a lateral cervical spine radiograph.

(c) The transverse ligament is anterior to the tectorial membrane and passes behind the dens.

(d) The apical ligament passes superiorly and inferiorly to the basiocciput and body of the axis, respectively, from the midpoint of the transverse ligament.

(e) Rotation of the head occurs at the atlanto-occipital joint.

(d) True – the arches unite first in the lumbar region and last in the cervical. The centrum unites first with the arch in the cervical region and in the lumbar region last.
(e) False – failure of fusion of the neural arches posteriorly results in spina bifida . Up to 20% of the population have defects in the lumbosacral region.

9.

(a) True
(b) False – the vertebral artery runs in a groove over the superior aspect of the posterior arch of the atlas. Between the groove and the lateral mass is the attachment for the posterior atlanto-occipital membrane, which may occasionally calcify laterally. This creates the arcuate foramen when the vertebral artery and sub-occipital nerve pass through.
(c) False – the axis (second cervical vertebrae) is the strongest of the cervical vertebrae.
(d) False – the tip of the dens develops from secondary centres at 3 years and fuses at 12 years. The dens unites with the rest of the body of the axis at 3 years.
(e) True – the dens has a lower signal intensity than the body on T_1-W MRI.

10.

(a) False – 2 mm in adults: 3 mm in children.
(b) True – on a lateral cervical spine radiograph, it is formed anteriorly by the pedicle and anterior body of axis; posteriorly by the vertebral body; superiorly by the upper margin of the superior articular facet; inferiorly by the inferior border of foramen transversarium.
(c) True – holds the median atlantoaxial joint.
(d) False – this is the cruciform ligament. The apical ligament passes from the dens to the anterior mid point of the foramen magnum.
(e) False – flexion, extension and lateral flexion take place at the atlanto-occipital joint. However, rotation occurs at the atlanto-axial joint around the vertical axis of the dens.

11. On a lateral cervical spine radiograph:

(a) No more than 15 mm of the dens should be above the Chamberlain's line.

(b) The anterior atlanto-axial distance should be less than 3 mm in adults in flexion-extension or in a neutral position.

(c) Tonsillar descent of 3–5 mm into the spinal canal is a normal feature.

(d) In adults from the atlas to the C4/5 disc the maximum dimension of the prevertebral soft tissue is 3 mm (with a film-target distance of 180 cm)

(e) On flexion and extension views, the offset from adjacent vertebrae seen in the posterior and anterior cortical margins, respectively, should not exceed 3 mm.

12. In the spine:

(a) The facet joints of the thoracic spine up to T10 are in the coronal plane and resist anterior translation.

(b) The 'collar of the Scotty dog' on an oblique radiograph of the lumbar spine is the pars interarticularis.

(c) The interpedicular distance increases progressively caudally.

(d) The articular facets of the lumbar vertebra face each other in the sagittal plane apart from the inferior facet of L5.

(e) Lumbarization of the first sacral segment is less common than sacralization of fifth lumbar vertebra.

13. The spinal cord:

(a) extends in the adult from foramen magnum to the first or second lumbar vertebra.

(b) segments differ by up to five in the lower thoracic region.

(c) tapers into the conus medullaris.

(d) has a lumbar expansion at the level of L1 to L5 vertebra.

(e) the anterior horns of the spinal cord contains the cell bodies of the motor neurones.

11.

(a) False – no more than a third of the dens or 5 mm of the dens should be above the Chamberlain's line. This line extends from the hard palate to the posterior lip of the foramen magnum. The McGregor line uses the inferior surface of the occiput rather than the foramen magnum.

(b) True – less than 5 mm in children, with a target to film distance of 180 cm.

(c) False – not in a lateral cervical radiograph, but in a midline sagittal MRI of the craniovertebral junction,tonsillar descent of 3–5 mm into the spinal canal is a normal feature.

(d) True – in children this may be up to 7 mm. Below this level the oesophagus increases the dimensions to up to 22 mm in adults, and in the lower cervical spine this dimension should not exceed that of the adjacent vertebral body.

(e) True

12.

(a) True

(b) True – the head is the transverse process, eye the pedicle, the ear is the superior articular process and the front limb of the 'dog' is the inferior articular facet, all of which belong to one vertebra.

(c) True

(d) True – this prevents forward translation on the sloping surface of the sacrum – L5 is an atypical vertebra.

(e) True – failure of segmentation at the lumbosacral level is seen in up to 6% of normal individuals.

13.

(a) True

(b) False – difference of one segment in lower cervical spine; two segments in upper thoracic and three in the lower thoracic.

(c) True

(d) False – from T10 to L1 vertebral levels the nerve roots emerge.

(e) True – posterior horns contain the cells of the sensory pathways.

14. In the spine:

(a) The first to the seventh cervical spinal nerves exit below the pedicle of the corresponding vertebrae.

(b) A postero-lateral prolapse of the L4/5 disc usually compresses the fifth lumbar root.

(c) The ventral and dorsal roots pass in front of and behind the denticulate ligament, respectively.

(d) The spinal dura mater is a continuation of the inner layer of the cerebral dura.

(e) The spinal dural sac is firmly attached to the anterior longitudinal ligament.

15. In the spine:

(a) The subarachnoid space contains about half the total volume of CSF.

(b) The pia mater is avascular.

(c) The three meningeal layers fuse with the periosteum of the first coccygeal segment.

(d) The filum terminale fuses with the periosteum of the first coccygeal segment.

(e) The dura is not seen on T_2 gradient echo images.

16. In the blood supply to the spinal cord:

(a) The anterior spinal artery is formed by the union of the anterior spinal branch of each vertebral artery.

(b) The anterior spinal artery supplies about two-thirds of the cord's cross-sectional area.

(c) Radicular arteries are branches of postero-lateral spinal arteries.

(d) The two posterior arteries supply the posterior white matter columns and the dorsal horns of the spinal cord.

(e) The main arterial supply to the lumbar enlargement is through the artery of Adamkiewicz.

14.

(a) False – there are eight cervical, twelve thoracic, five lumbar, five sacral and one coccygeal segmental nerves. The first to the seventh cervical spinal nerves exit above the pedicle of the corresponding vertebrae, whereas all the other roots exit below the pedicles.

(b) False – fourth lumbar root. However, a similar situation in the cervical vertebra would compress the fifth cervical root.

(c) True

(d) True – the epidural (extradural) space is between the periosteum of the vertebrae (which represents the outer periosteal layer of the dura) and the spinal dura mater.

(e) False – it is attached to the tectorial membrane and posterior longitudinal ligament.

15.

(a) True – 75 ml out of the total 150 ml.

(b) False – the pia mater is applied to the surface of the spinal cord and is vascular.

(c) True

(d) True

(e) False

16.

(a) True – runs in the anterior median fissure.

(b) True

(c) False – in the cervical region, they usually arise from branches of vertebral, deep cervical arteries, costocervical trunk or rarely from the thyrocervical branch of the subclavian. In the thoracic region they are branches of the supreme intercostal arteries and the aortic intercostal arteries.

(d) True

(e) True – also known as the arteria radicularis magna, this artery usually arises between T9 and L1 segments, from the tenth or eleventh thoracic radicular arteries. However, its origin is inconstant and paraplegia may result as a complication of aortography due to varying amounts of contrast medium being directed towards the spinal arteries via the lumbar arteries, particularly in aortic stenosis.

Index